CBS Confident Pharmacy Series

Pharmaceutical Chemistry I

Third Edition

for First Year Diploma in Pharmacy

(0806) Strictly Based on Syllabus as per ER1991

Question–Answer Type Notes and **Board Question Papers** (1996 to 2017)

Salient Features

- Total Confidence and 100 percent Success in Every Examination.
- Repeatedly Asked Board Questions Indicated in Brackets.
- Chapterwise Collection of Very Important Questions.
- Written in Very Simple and Lucid Language.
- Board Question Papers 2015–2017 given at the End of Text.

CBS Titles by the same Author in

CBS Confident Pharmacy Series

First Year D Pharm

1. Pharmaceutics I, 3/e
2. Pharmaceutical Chemistry I, 3/e
3. Pharmacognosy, 3/e
4. Biochemistry and Clinical Pathology, 3/e
5. Human Anatomy and Physiology, 3/e
6. Health Education and Community Pharmacy, 3/e

Second Year D Pharm

1. Pharmaceutics II, 3/e
2. Pharmaceutical Chemistry II, 3/e
3. Pharmacology and Toxicology, 3/e
4. Pharmaceutical Jurisprudence, 3/e
5. Drug Store and Business Management, 3/e
6. Hospital and Clinical Pharmacy, 3/e

CBS Confident Pharmacy Series

Pharmaceutical Chemistry I

Third Edition

for First Year Diploma in Pharmacy
(**0806**) Strictly Based on Syllabus as per ER1991

V.N. Raje M Pharm

Principal
Gourishankar Education Society's
GES College of Pharmacy (D Pharm)
Limb, Satara, Maharashtra

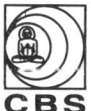

CBS Publishers & Distributors Pvt Ltd

New Delhi • Bengaluru • Chennai • Kochi • Kolkata • Mumbai
Hyderabad • Jharkhand • Nagpur • Patna • Pune • Uttarakhand

Pharmaceutical Chemistry I
Third Edition

Disclaimer

Science and technology are constantly changing fields. New research and experience broaden the scope of information and knowledge. The author has tried his best in giving information available to him while preparing the material for this book. Although, all efforts have been made to ensure optimum accuracy of the material, yet it is quite possible some errors might have been left uncorrected. The publisher, the printer and the author will not be held responsible for any inadvertent errors or inaccuracies.

ISBN: 978-93-86478-64-1

Copyright © Author and Publisher

Third Edition: 2018
Reprint: 2018, 2019, 2020, 2021
First Edition: 2010
Reprint: 2011
Second Edition: 2015
Reprint: 2016

All rights reserved. No part of this book may be reproduced or transmitted in any form or by any means, electronic or mechanical, including photocopying, recording, or any information storage and retrieval system without permission, in writing, from the author and the publisher.

Published by Satish Kumar Jain and produced by Varun Jain for

CBS Publishers & Distributors Pvt Ltd

4819/XI Prahlad Street, 24 Ansari Road, Daryaganj, New Delhi 110 002, India.
Ph: 011-23289259, 23266861, 23266867 Website: www.cbspd.com
Fax: 011-23243014 e-mail: delhi@cbspd.com; cbspubs@airtelmail.in.
Corporate Office: 204 FIE, Industrial Area, Patparganj, Delhi 110 092
Ph: 011-4934 4934 Fax: 011-4934 4935 e-mail: publishing@cbspd.com; publicity@cbspd.com

Branches

- **Bengaluru:** Seema House 2975, 17th Cross, K.R. Road, Banasankari 2nd Stage, Bengaluru 560 070, Karnataka
  Ph: +91-80-26771678/79 Fax: +91-80-26771680 e-mail: bangalore@cbspd.com
- **Chennai:** 7, Subbaraya Street, Shenoy Nagar, Chennai 600 030, Tamil Nadu
  Ph: +91-44-26680620, 26681266 Fax: +91-44-42032115 e-mail: chennai@cbspd.com
- **Kochi:** 42/1325, 1326 Power House Road, Opp. KSEB, Kochi 682018, Kerala
  Ph: +91-484-4059061-65 Fax: +91-484-4059065 e-mail: kochi@cbspd.com
- **Kolkata:** 6/B, Ground Floor, Rameswar Shaw Road, Kolkata-700 014, West Bengal
  Ph: +91-33-22891126, 22891127, 22891128 e-mail: kolkata@cbspd.com
- **Mumbai:** 83-C, Dr E Moses Road, Worli, Mumbai-400018, Maharashtra
  Ph: +91-22-24902340/41 Fax: +91-22-24902342 e-mail: mumbai@cbspd.com

Representatives

- **Hyderabad** 0-9885175004
- **Jharkhand** 0-9811541605
- **Nagpur** 0-9421945513
- **Patna** 0-9334159340
- **Pune** 0-9623451994
- **Uttarakhand** 0-9716462459

Printed at Mudrak, Noida, UP, India

to
my beloved family

Preface to the Third Edition

The Third edition of the now popular and successful book includes Board Question Papers 1996 to 2017. The book has been written to meet the requirements of students of Diploma in Pharmacy (D Pharm) in accordance with the new revised syllabus ER1991 prescribed by Pharmacy Council of India.

This book is small and humble effort has been put in for compiling necessary information on the subject. An attempt has been made to demystify and simplify the basic concepts for the students of pharmacy and to enable them get an evergreen success in MSBTE examinations.

The salient features of the present book are:

- Lucid and easy language
- To the point answers
- Remembering facts in the simplest way
- Infusing confidence in the reader to appear in the Board Examinations.

Hence the series is named

CBS Confident Pharmacy Series

I am confident that this book will be useful to both the students and the teachers of Diploma in Pharmacy as well as the candidates desiring to succeed in competitive examinations for better job opportunities in pharmacy profession such as hospital pharmacists in PHCs, civil hospitals, etc.

Raje Vijay N

Acknowledgements

I express my heartfelt thanks to Prof Madan Jagtap, Chairman, Gourishankar Education Society, Satara Maharashtra, for consistent encouragement and inspiration for writing this book.

I wish to acknowledge the prompt and efficient help given by Prof Milind Jagtap, Mr Jaywant Salunkhe, Mr Appa Rajage, Mr Nitin Mudalgikar, and Mr Shrirang Katekar of Gourishankar Education Society, Satara.

I am also thankful to Shri Satish Kumar Jain, Chairman and Managing Director, and Shri RN Mandal, General Manager, Pune Branch, CBS Publishers & Distributors Pvt Ltd, for their sustained efforts and keen interest in the publication of this book.

I wish all my beloved students to have a great success in the Board Examinations.

Raje Vijay N

Syllabus
(As per ER 1991)

Pharmaceutical Chemistry I

- General discussion on the following inorganic compounds including important physical and chemical properties, medicinal and pharmaceutical uses storage condition and chemical incompatibility.
  i. **Acids, Bases and Buffers:** Boric acid*, Hydrochloric acid, Strong ammonium hydroxide, Calcium hydroxide, Sodium hydroxide and official buffers.
  ii. **Antioxidants:** Hypophosphorous acid, Sulphur dioxide, Sodium bisulfphite, Sodium meta-bisulphite, Sodium thiosulphate, Nitrogen and Sodium nitrite.
  iii. **Gastrointestinal Agents:**
      a. **Acidifying agents:** Dilute hydrochloric acid.
      b. **Antacids:** Sodium bicarbonate, Aluminium hydroxide gel, Aluminium phosphate, Calcium carbonate, Magnesium carbonate, Magnesium trisilicate, Magnesium oxide, Combination of antacid preparations.
      c. **Protectives and absorbents:** Bismuth subcarbonate and Kaolin.
      d. **Saline cathartics:** Sodium potassium tartrate and magnesium sulphate.
  iv. **Topical Agents:**
      a. **Protectives:** Talc, Zinc oxide, Calamine, Zinc stearate, Titanium dioxide, Silicone polymers.
      b. **Antimicrobials and astringents:** Hydrogen peroxide; Potassium povidone-iodine, Boric acid, Borax, Silver nitrate, Mild silver protein, Mercury, Yellow mercuric oxide, Ammoniated mercury.
      c. **Sulphur and its compounds:** Sublimed sulphur, Precipitated sulphur, Selenium sulphide.

x Pharmaceutical Chemistry I

d. **Astringents:** Alum and zinc sulphate.
e. **Dental products:** Sodium fluoride, stannous fluoride, calcium carbonate, sodium meta phosphate, dicalcium phosphate, strontium chloride, zinc chloride.
f. **Inhalants:** Oxygen, carbon dioxide, nitrous oxide.
g. **Respiratory stimulants:** Ammonium carbonate.
h. **Expectorants and emetics:** Ammonium chloride*, potassium iodide, Antimony potassium tartrate.
i. **Antidotes:** Sodium nitrate.

- **Major Intra-Extracellular Electrolytes**
  i. Electrolytes used for replacement therapy: Sodium chloride and its preparations, potassium chloride and its preparations.
  ii. Physiological acid–base balance and electorates used: Sodium acetate, potassium acetate, sodium bicarbonate infection, sodium citrate, potassium citrate, sodium lactate infection, ammonium chloride and its injection.
  iii. Combination of oral electrolytes powders and solutions.

- Inorganic Official Compounds of Iron, Iodine and Calcium, Ferrous sulphate and Calcium gluconate.

- **Radiopharmaceutical and Contrast Media:** Radioactivity, Alpha, Beta and Gamma radiations, Biological effects of radiations, Measurements of radioactivity, GM counter—Radio isotopes—their uses, storage and precautions with Special Reference to the Official Preparations.

Radiopaque Contrast Media—Barium Sulphate

- **Quality Control of Drugs and Pharmaceutical:** Importance of Quality Control, Significant Errors, Methods used for Quality Control, Sources of Impurities in Pharmaceuticals. Limit Tests for Arsenic, chloride, Sulphate Iron and Heavy Metals.

Identification Tests for Cations and Anions as per Indian Pharmacopoeia.

Contents

Preface to the Third Edition .... *vii*

1. Definitions 1
2. Acids, Bases and Buffers 7
3. Antioxidants 14
4. Gastrointestinal Agents 18
5. Topical Agents 27
6. Dental Products 38
7. Inhalants 42
8. Respiratory Stimulants 45
9. Expectorants and Emetics 47
10. Antidotes 50
11. Electrolytes 52
12. Official Compounds of Iodine, Iron and Calcium 59
13. Radioactivity 62
14. Quality Control of Drugs and Pharmaceuticals 69

    Board Question Papers *83*

1

Definitions

1. **Acid:** A substance which gives hydronium ions (H^+) in aqueous solution is called acid, e.g. dilute HCl, dilute HNO_3, H_2SO_4.
2. **Base:** A substance which gives hydroxyl ions (OH^-) in aqueous solution is called base, e.g. KOH, NaOH, $Ca(OH)_2$.
3. **Buffers/buffer solutions:** A solution which resists the changes in pH upon the addition of a small amount of acid or alkali.
4. **Buffer capacity:** It is defined as the moles of strong acid or strong base required to change the pH of 1 litre of the buffer solution by 1 unit.
5. **Antioxidants:** The substances which can prevent the oxidation of other materials are called antioxidants, e.g. sodium nitrite, SO_2.
6. **Gastrointestinal agents:** The drugs which are used in the treatment of various gastrointestinal disorders are called GIT agents.
7. **Acidifying agents:** The substances which increase the level of acid in the stomach are called acidifying agents, e.g. dilute HCl.
8. **Achlorhydria:** It means absence of hydrochloric acid in the stomach.
9. **Hypochlorhydria:** It means decrease in secretion of dilute HCl in the stomach below the normal level.
10. **Antacids:** The substances which neutralize excessive or abnormal acidity in the stomach are called antacids, e.g. sodium bicarbonate, magnesium hydroxide, aluminium hydroxide gel.
11. **Protectives:** These are the substances which protect the exposed surface from harmful stimuli, e.g. kaolin, bismuth carbonate.

12. **Adsorbants:** The substances which are used to absorb the gases, toxins and bacteria are called adsorbants, e.g. kaolin, activated charcoal.
13. **Saline cathartics/purgatives:** The drugs which increase the removal of materials from the intestine are called saline cathartics, e.g. magnesium sulphate, sodium sulphate.
14. **Topical agents:** The agents which are applied topically or locally to the skin or mucus membranes are called topical agents, e.g. calamine, iodine, castor oil.
15. **Astringents:** The substances which cause precipitation of superficial proteins are called astringents, e.g. alum, zinc sulphate.
16. **Antimicrobial agents:** The agents which are used to kill the microbes are called antimicrobial agents, e.g. hydrogen peroxide, boric acid, iodine.
17. **Antiseptics:** The drugs that prevent sepsis are called antiseptics, e.g. iodine, H_2O_2.
18. **Disinfectants:** The substances that prevent the infection by destroying the pathogenic microorganisms are called disinfectants.
19. **Germicides:** The agents which kill the germs are called germicides.
20. **Bactericides:** The agents which kill the bacteria are called bactericides.
21. **Bacteriostatics:** The agents which stop the growth of bacteria.
22. **Scabicides:** The agents which are used in the treatment of scabies.
23. **Topical protectives:** The substances which are applied on the skin for protection are called topical protectives, e.g. talc, calamine, zinc oxide, zinc stearate.
24. **Dental products:** The preparations which are used for the treatment of various dental disorders are called dental products.
25. **Dental caries/tooth decay:** It is a disease of teeth characterized by decalcification and gives bad odour of the mouth.
26. **Anticaries agents:** The agents which are used in the treatment of dental caries/tooth decay are called anticaries agents, e.g. sodium fluoride, stannous fluoride.

27. **Cleansing agents/abrasives:** The substances which are used to remove stain from the teeth are called cleansing agents, e.g. calcium phosphate, dicalcium phosphate, sodium phosphate.
28. **Polishing agents:** The substances which give whiteness to teeth by their abrasive action are called polishing agents, e.g. stannous fluoride, calcium carbonate.
29. **Desensitizing agents:** The substances which reduce the sensitivity of teeth to heat and cold are known as desensitizing agents, e.g. zinc chloride, strontium chloride.
30. **Dentifrices:** The substances which are used for cleansing dirty surface of the tooth are called dentifrices, e.g. calcium phosphate, calcium carbonate.
31. **Dental fluorosis:** When more quantity of fluoride is ingested, it is carried to bones and teeth and produce mottling of enamel which is known as dental fluorosis.
32. **Inhalants:** The substances which are in vapour or gas form are inhaled through nose are called inhalants, e.g. O_2, N_2O, CO_2.
33. **Respiratory stimulants:** The substances which stimulate the rate of respiration are called respiratory stimulants, e.g. ammonium carbonate.
34. **Expectorants:** The substances which remove the sputums from the respiratory tract are called expectorants, e.g. ammonium chloride, potassium iodide.
35. **Emetics:** The substances which produce vomiting are called emetics, e.g. antimony potassium tartrate, copper sulphate.
36. **Antidotes:** The agents which stop the actions of poison are called antidotes, e.g. sodium nitrite, sodium thiosulphate.
37. **Electrolytes:** The substances whose aqueous solutions conduct electricity are known as electrolytes.
38. **Intracellular fluid/ICF:** It is the fluid present in the cell, e.g. cytoplasm.
39. **Extracellular fluid/ECF:** It is the fluid present outside the cell, e.g. tissue fluid.
40. **Plasma fluid:** It is the fluid present within the blood, e.g. blood plasma.

41. **Replacement therapy:** The external administration of electrolytes in the body to correct electrolyte balance of the body is known as replacement therapy.
42. **Electrolyte replenishers:** The substances which are used to correct body fluid electrolyte balance are called electrolyte replenishers.
43. **ORS/ORT:** The preparations which are given orally to correct electrolyte balance of the body are called oral rehydration salts (ORS) and therapy is called oral rehydration therapy (ORT).
44. **Hypokalemia:** It means decreased level of potassium in the blood.
45. **Hyperkalemia:** It means increased level of potassium in the blood.
46. **Hyponatremia:** It means decreased level of sodium in the blood.
47. **Hypernatremia:** It means increased level of sodium in the blood.
48. **Haematinics:** The substances which increase the amount of haemoglobin in the blood are called haematinics, e.g. ferrous sulphate, ferrous gluconate, vitamin B_{12}.
49. **Radioactivity:** It is the spontaneous and continuous emission of α, β and γ radiations from the substance.
50. **Radiopharmaceuticals/radioactive substances:** The substances which emit radioactive radiations and are used in medicine are called radiopharmaceuticals/radioactive substances, e.g. calcium (Ca^{44} and Ca^{45}), carbon (C^{14}), cobalt (Co^{60}).
51. **Radiopaque contrast media/X-ray contrast media:** The substances which have a capacity to prevent passage of X-ray and hence appear opaque on X-ray examination are called radiopaque substances.

    The medium which gives this type of effect is called X-ray contrast medium, e.g. barium sulphate, iodine compounds, bismuth compounds.
52. **Half-life:** It is the time in which the amount of radioactive substance is decreased to ½ of its original.

$$t_{1/2} = \frac{0.693}{\lambda}, \lambda = \text{decay constant}$$

53. **Nuclide:** Nuclide is a species of atom characterized by the constitution of the nucleus, in particular by the number of protons and neutrons in the nucleus.

54. **Isotopes:** The species which have different atomic mass number but the same atomic number are called isotopes, e.g.

$$^{206}_{82}Pb, \; ^{207}_{82}Pb \; ^{208}_{82}Pb$$

55. **Isobars:** The atoms of different elements having different atomic numbers and same atomic mass numbers are called isobars, e.g.

$$^{14}_{6}C \; \& \; ^{14}_{7}N$$

56. **Isotones:** Atomic species having same number of neutrons but different mass numbers are called isotones.

57. **Nuclear isomers:** Atoms of the same elements having same atomic number and same atomic mass number but differ in radioactive properties are called nuclear isomers.

58. **Curie:** It is the quantity of any radioactive substance undergoing the same number of disintegrations in unit time as that of 1 gm of radium.

59. **Rad:** It is defined as the quantity of radiation which releases or absorbs 100 erg/gm of specified medium.

60. **Roentgen:** It is the unit of measurement of ionising effect of radiation by measuring damaging effect on biological matter.

61. **Quality control:** It is a day-to-day process of controlling quality of every incoming material till the finished product quality.

62. **Quality assurance:** Quality assurance is the department which includes a total quality control, government regulations, company standard and development of standard operating procedures of analysis.

63. **Significant figures:** Significant figures can be defined as the number of digits necessary to express the results of a measurement consistent with the measured precision.

64. **Impurity:** Impurity is the undesirable material which may or may not be toxic, present in pharmaceutical substances.

65. **Limit tests:** Limit tests are the qualitative tests used to identify the small amounts of impurities present in the substance.

66. **Tests for purity:** These are the tests used for detecting impurities in the pharmaceutical substances.
67. **Ash:** Ash is the residue after complete ignition of the drug.
68. **LOD:** It means loss of drying of the substance.
69. **LOI:** It means loss of ignition of the substance.
70. **Pharmacopoeia:** It is an official book of standards published by respective governments containing list of drugs, pharmaceuticals, uses, preparations, storage, etc.
71. **Assay:** The estimation of active principle present in a drug or pharmaceutical is known as assay.
72. **Monograph of a drug:** It means detail study of drug with reference to title, synonym, preparations, storage category, official preparation, etc.
73. **Normal solution:** A solution containing 1 gm equivalent weight per thousand ml of solution.
74. **Molar solution:** A solution containing 1 mole per thousand ml of solution.

2

Acids, Bases and Buffers

Q 1. Define acid and base as per different theories.

According to Lewis Concept (W. 03, 08)

Acid

The substance which can accept the lone pair of electrons is called acid, e.g. HCl, H_2SO_4.

Base

The substance which can donate the lone pair of electrons is called base, e.g. NaOH, KOH.

According to Arrehenious Theory (S. 99, 00, 05; W. 06, 07)

Acid

The substance which gives hydrogen (H^+) ion in water is called acid.

Base

The substance which gives hydroxyl (OH^-) ion in water is called base.

According to Lowry and Bronsted Theory (S. 04, 06, 07; W. 99, 00, 01, 02)

Acid

The substance which can donate the protons to the solution is called acid.

Base

The substance which can accept the protons is called base.

Q 2. What are buffer solutions? Give the types of buffers. (S. 97, 00, 02, 03; W. 96, 97, 01, 02, 05)

Buffer Solutions

The solutions which resist the changes in pH upon the addition of small amount of acid or alkali are called buffer solutions.

Types/Classification of Buffers

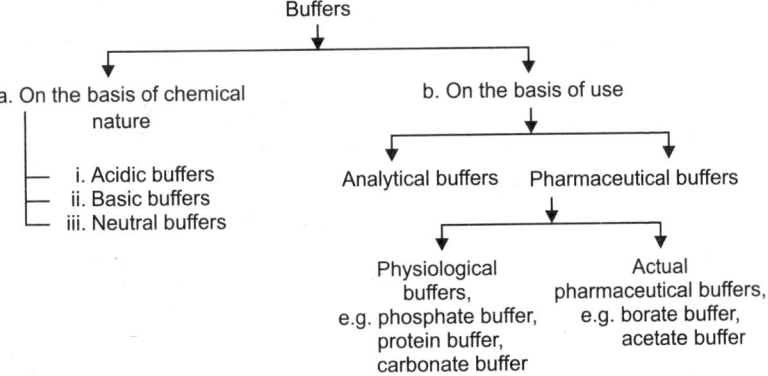

- *Acidic buffer*: It is a combination of weak acid and its corresponding salt, e.g. mixture of acetic acid and sodium acetate.
- *Basic buffer*: It is a combination of weak base and its corresponding salt, e.g. mixture of ammonium hydroxide and ammonium chloride.
- *Neutral buffer*: It is a single substance showing the properties of buffer, e.g. ammonium acetate.

Q 3. Define buffer capacity. Give the properties of buffer solutions. (S. 01, 09; W. 01, 07, 08)

Buffer Capacity

It is defined as the moles of strong acid or strong base required to change the pH of 1 litre of the solution by 1 unit.

Properties of Buffer

- The pH of buffer solution is constant.
- The pH of solution does not change on dilution.
- The pH does not change even after addition of small quantities of acids or bases.
- As the pH of buffer solution is constant, it is useful in a number of chemical reactions.

Acids, Bases and Buffers 9

Q 4. What factors should be considered during selection of a suitable buffer?

For selection of buffer, chemical factors and pharmacological factors must be considered.

Chemical Factors
- The buffer system should not react with other chemicals in the preparation.
- The buffer system should have reasonable chemical stability.
- Buffer capacity depends on absolute concentration of each buffer compound.

Pharmaceutical Factors
- *Toxicity of buffers*: Some of the buffers have limited use in pharmaceutical practice because of their toxicity.
- *Effect or pharmacological action of the preparation*: Buffer system should not interact with action of ingredients of preparation.
- *Contamination by microorganisms*: Many buffer systems support microbial growth as they can serve as nutrient media for moulds and microorganisms particularly when the pH is close to neutrality.

Q 5. Explain the role of buffers in pharmacy. (S. 99, 09; W. 00, 04, 06)

Buffers are used to provide a specific pH for analytical purposes as well as to maintain pH of drug preparations.
The buffer systems which cover the pH range from 1.2 to 10 are as follows:
  i. *Hydrochloric acid buffer*: (pH 1.2–2.2 in 0.1 unit intervals)
  ii. *Acid phthalate buffer*: (pH 2.2–4.0 in 0.2 unit intervals)
  iii. *Neutralised phthalate buffer*: (pH 4.2–5.8 in 0.2 unit intervals)
  iv. *Phosphate buffer*: (pH 5.8–8.0 in 0.2 unit intervals)
  v. *Alkaline borate buffer*: (pH 8.0–10 in 0.2 unit intervals).

Role of Buffers in Pharmacy

The buffers are important in pharmaceutical preparations to ensure stable pH conditions for the medicinally active compounds.
- Solubility of many compounds is controlled by providing a suitable pH.
- Colour of many compounds is pH-dependant.
- pH gives stability of different preparations.

- It provides patient comfort.
- Citric acid is used for stabilising milk of magnesia.
- Penicillin preparations are stabilised by addition of carbonates.
- Sulphonamide preparations are stabilised by addition of sodium bicarbonate, sodium acetate or sodium citrate.

Q 6. Distinguish between phosphate buffer and borate buffer.

Phosphate buffer	Borate buffer
i. It is composed of monohydrogen and dihydrogen phosphate.	i. It consists of tetraborate ion and boric acid.
ii. pKa is 7.2.	ii. pKa is 9.2.
iii. It is non-toxic.	iii. Toxic, if taken internally.
iv. It is useful for internal preparations and parenteral preparations.	iv. It is generally used for external preparations only.

Q 7. Write a note on "phosphate buffer".

- It is composed of monohydrogen and dihydrogen phosphate.
- The acidic member of this buffer is dihydrogen phosphate while basic member is monohydrogen phosphate.
- The pKa of acidic member is reasonably closed to the pH of blood. Thus, it is one of the physiological buffers.
- pKa of phosphate buffer is 7.2.
- It is used for ophthalmic preparations, parenteral preparations and internal preparations.

Advantages of Phosphate Buffer

- It is nontoxic, therefore, useful for internal preparations and parenteral preparations.
- Useful for ophthalmic preparations.
- pKa of dihydrogen phosphate is 7.2, i.e. closed to pH of blood.

Disadvantages of Phosphate Buffer

- Incompatible with Zn, Al salts because these salts are insoluble in buffer.
- It can support microbial growth, therefore, preservative is needed.

Q 8. Write a note on "borate buffer".

It consists of tetraborate ion and boric acid.

Advantages

- It is generally used for external preparation only.
- These buffers cover the pH range from 7 to 11.
- It is used for ophthalmic, nasal and ear preparations.
- It is an antimicrobial only in powder form.

Disadvantages

- It is toxic, if taken internally, therefore, not useful for oral and parenteral preparations.
- pKa of boric acid is 9.2 which is not efficient at physiological pH.
- It is susceptible for microbial growth in liquid form, therefore, preservative like benzalkonium chloride is needed.

Q 9. Write a note on (a) boric acid, (b) sodium hydroxide, (c) strong ammonium hydroxide, (d) calcium hydroxide, (e) strong ammonia solution.

(a) **Boric Acid IP (S. 97, 00, 03, 09; W. 96, 97))**

- *Synonym*: Orthoboric acid
- *Formula*: H_3BO_3
- *Properties*
  i. It is a white, odourless powder with bitter taste.
  ii. It is soapy to touch.
  iii. Soluble in hot water and freely soluble in glycerine.
  iv. Solution is isotonic with body fluids.
- *Storage:* It should be stored in well closed container. Label should indicate:
  "It should not be taken internally."
  "It should not be applied on broken skin."
- *Incompatibility:* It is incompatible with tannins.
- *Uses*
  i. Externally for irrigation of organs
  ii. Cleaning of wounds
  iii. Mild antiseptic
  iv. In dusting powders
  v. Ingredient of mouthwash and eyewash
  vi. Buffer in ophthalmic preparations
  vii. To reduce inflammation of various skin disorders.

(b) Sodium Hydroxide (S. 97, 04, 07; W. 97, 98, 99, 04)
- *Synonym*: Caustic soda
- *Formula*: NaOH
- *Properties*
  i. White odourless salt
  ii. Available in pellets form
  iii. Soluble in water and alcohol
  iv. It is a very strong base.
- *Storage*: It is stored in tightly closed container as it absorbs moisture and carbon dioxide.
- *Uses*
  i. As a laboratory reagent.
  ii. In the preparation of soap.

(c) Strong Ammonium Hydroxide
- *Synonym*: Strong ammonia solution, liquor ammonia fortis.
- *Formula*: NH_4OH
- *Properties*
  i. It is a colourless liquid with pungent odour.
  ii. Alkaline in taste.
  iii. Miscible with water.
  iv. Reacts with metal to form nitrogen gas.
- *Storage*: In a tightly closed container in cool place.
  Label: "Handle with care", "Do not taste", "Avoid inhalation of vapours".
- *Uses*
  i. As a source of ammonia.
  ii. Antacid.
  iii. Counterirritant and respiratory stimulant.
  iv. As a fertilizer.
  v. In preparations of aromatic spirit of ammonia.
  vi. As a laboratory reagent.

(d) Calcium Hydroxide (S. 09)
- *Synonym*: Slaked lime or hydrated lime.
- *Formula*: $Ca(OH)_2$.
- *Properties*:
  i. White soft powder.
  ii. Bitter in taste.

Acids, Bases and Buffers 13

   iii. Slightly soluble in water.
   iv. Insoluble in alcohol.
   v. Aqueous suspension is alkaline to litmus.
- *Storage*: It should be kept in tightly closed containers protected from moisture.
- *Incompatibility*: Incompatible with CO_2.
- *Uses*
    i. As a source of calcium.
   ii. As antacid.
  iii. As electrolyte replenisher.
   iv. Astringent in diarrhoea.
    v. Emulsifying agent in soap formation.
   vi. As ingredient of ointment and skin lotions.

(e) **Strong Ammonia Solution (S. 97, 09; W. 97, 01, 04, 05, 08)**
- *Formula*: NH_3
- *Properties*
    i. It is clear, colourless liquid having an exceeding pungent, characteristic odour.
   ii. Its specific gravity is about 0.90.
- *Caution*: Strong ammonia solution should be handled carefully because of its caustic nature of solution and irritating properties of vapours. Cool the container well before opening and cover the closure with a cloth or other material while opening.
  Do not taste strong ammonia solution and avoid inhalation of its vapours.
- *Storage*: Preserve ammonia solution (strong) in a well closed container in a cool place.
- *Medicinal and pharmaceutical uses*
    i. Its salts are used as an antacid, counter irritant and respiratory stimulant.
   ii. Dilute solution of ammonia (10%) is a common reagent and a basc.

3

Antioxidants

Q 1. What are antioxidants? Classify antioxidants with examples. Give ideal properties. OR Write a note/brief account of antioxidants. (S. 96, 97, 00, 01, 02, 03, 07, 08; W. 96, 97, 98, 99, 00, 01, 04, 05, 06, 07, 08)

Antioxidants

The substances which prevent the oxidation of medicinally active compounds are called antioxidants.
Antioxidants are used to prevent rancidity of oils and fats or deterioration of materials due to oxidation.

Classification

- *Organic antioxidants*: Tocopherols, phenols, parabens, gallic acid.
- *Inorganic antioxidants*: Sulphur dioxide, nitrogen, sodium nitrite, hypophosphoric acid, sodium metabisulphate.

Mechanism of Action

- *Organic antioxidants*: They have antimicrobial property. They can prevent spoilage of product which is due to antimicrobial action.
- *Inorganic antioxidants*: Inorganic antioxidants act as reducing agents.
  They prevent oxidation and get oxidised themselves.

$$\text{oxidation} + e \rightleftharpoons \text{reduction}$$

Ideal Requirement of an Antioxidant

- It should prevent the oxidation of product.
- It should be effective in low concentration.
- It should be stable.
- It should be nontoxic and nonirritant.
- It should not cause allergic reactions.

Antioxidants   15

- It should not affect the colour, odour and taste of the preparation.
- It should be compatible with ingredients, closure and container.
- It should be physiologically inert.

Q 2. Write a note on gaseous antioxidants.

These are used to prevent oxidation of generally liquid preparation, e.g. sulphur dioxide (SO_2), nitrogen (N_2). The air present in the containers contains oxygen which oxidises the medicinally active compound present in that liquid. Therefore, to avoid the oxidation of medicinally active substances from the oxygen, the air containing oxygen is replaced by environment of N_2 and SO_2 in empty containers. Further, the containers are filled and sealed in the environment of inorganic antioxidants. Some examples are as follows:

a. **Sulphur Dioxide (SO_2) (W. 97)**
- *Preparation*: It is prepared by burning of sulphur in presence of air.
$$2\,S + O_2 \longrightarrow SO_2$$
- *Properties*
  i. It is a colourless, noninflammable gas.
  ii. Characteristic pungent odour.
  iii. Its aqueous solution is acidic to litmus.
  iv. Miscible with H_2O.
- *Storage*: It is stored in strong metallic cylinders.
- *Incompatibility*: It is incompatible with oxidising agent.
- *Uses*
  i. Antioxidant.
  ii. As a stabilizer in soft drinks.
  iii. Used in refrigerator.
  iv. In fermentation.
  v. With glycerin, it is used in treatment of tonsilitis.

b. **Nitrogen (N_2) (W. 96, 98, 05)**
- *Properties*
  i. It is a colourless, odourless gas.
  ii. Miscible with water.
  iii. Noninflammable.
  iv. It is an inert gas.

- *Storage*: It is stored in black-painted airtight cylinder.
- *Uses*
  i. Used as an antioxidant for preservation of liquid dosage forms.
  ii. Used to replace air in containers for parenterals and solutions for topical application.
  iii. Nitrogen is also used to retard oxidation in the qualitative test for carbon monoxide.

Q 3. Describe in brief (a) hypophosphorus acid, (b) sodium metabisulphate, (c) sodium thiosulphate.

(a) **Hypophosphorus Acid (W. 08)**
- *Formula*: H_3PO_2
- *Properties*
  i. It is a clear, colourless liquid.
  ii. Soluble in water and alcohol.
  iii. Its aqueous solution is acidic to litmus.
  iv. It is slightly yellowish in colour.
- *Storage*: It should be stored in well closed light-resistant container.
- *Incompatibility*: With oxidising agents, heavy metals, lead, mercury.
- *Uses*
  i. In syrup preparation as antioxidant.
  ii. In table formulation.
  iii. As a laboratory agent.
  iv. To avoid the formation of free iodine in dilute hydroiodic acid.

(b) **Sodium Metabisulphate (S. 00, 03; W. 96, 97, 98, 99)**
- *Formula*: $Na_2S_2O_5$
- *Synonym*: Disodium pyrosulphide.
- *Properties*
  i. White to yellowish white powder.
  ii. Tasteless.
  iii. Having characteristic odour of sulphur.
  iv. Freely soluble in water, slightly soluble in alcohol.
  v. It becomes yellow on storage.
- *Storage*: It should be stored in a tightly-closed containers
- *Incompatibility*: With oxidising agents, with chloramphenicol.

- *Uses*
    i. As antioxidant.
    ii. As a food preservative.
    iii. In treatment of skin diseases.
    iv. As a stabilizer in many injections.

(c) **Sodium Thiosulphate (S. 97, 00, 09; W. 96, 97, 98, 99, 01, 08)**
- *Formula*: $Na_2S_2O_3 \cdot 5H_2O$
- *Properties*
    i. Colourless, transparent crystals.
    ii. Soluble in water, insoluble in alcohol.
    iii. It has cooling and bitter taste.
- *Storage*: It should be stored in tightly-closed light-resistant container.
- *Incompatibility*: With oxidising agents.
- *Uses*
    i. Antioxidant.
    ii. Antidote.
    iii. In treatment of iodine toxicity.
    iv. In skin disorders.
    v. As laboratory agent.

4

Gastrointestinal Agents

Q 1. What are GIT agents? Classify gastrointestinal agents with examples. Classify inorganic compounds acting as gastrointestinal agents. (S. 00, 01, 02; W. 96, 98, 99, 00, 02, 05)

GIT Agents

The agents which are used to treat gastrointestinal disorders are called gastrointestinal agents.

Classification

- *Acidifying agents*: Dilute HCl.
- *Antacids*: Sodium bicarbonate, aluminium hydroxide gel, calcium carbonate, magnesium trisillicate, magnesium oxide, magnesium carbonate.
- *Protective and adsorbents*: Bismuth subcarbonate, bismuth subgallate, milk of bismuth, kaolin.
- *Saline cathartics* (purgatives/laxatives): Magnesium sulphate, sodium potassium tartrate.

Q 2. Write a note on "acidifying agents". (S. 96, 00, 01)

Acidifying Agents

These substances which increase the acidity in stomach are called acidifying agents.

Mechanism of Action

These substances increase the acidity in stomach by one of the following mechanisms:
  i. They increase acidic concentration due to acidic nature.
  ii. They increase the acidity in stomach by stimulating the secretory cells of GIT.

Gastrointestinal Agents 19

Types of Acidifying Agents

- Inorganic acidifying agents increase the acidity because they are acidic in nature, e.g. dilute HCl.
- Organic acidifying agents act by increasing the secretion of gastric acid, e.g. glutamic acid.

Explanation

The epithelial cells of gastric mucosa secrete the endogenous HCl and required enzymes which are necessary for digestion. Acidic drugs are mostly absorbed from stomach. If acidic concentration is below 4.5 pH, only activity of pepsin is observed. Pepsin is active at pH range 3.5–5. If secretion of gastric acid is decreased normal condition is called "hypochlorhydria". If secretion of gastric acid is totally absent, it is called "achlorhydria."

Symptoms of Achlorhydria

Abdominal pains, loss of appetite, mild diarrhoea, confusion.

Q 3. Explain the term "achlorhydria". Write a note on drug used in the treatment of achlorhydria/monograph of dilute HCl. (S. 99, 00, 02, 03, 05, 06, 08; W. 98, 99, 00)

Achlorhydria

When the secretion of gastric acid is totally absent, the condition is called achlorhydria.

Symptoms

- Abdominal pains.
- Loss of appetite.
- Mild diarrhoea.
- Confusion.

Dilute HCl

- *Standard*: It contains 10% w/w of HCl.
- *Properties*
    i. It is a clear, colourless, tasteless, odourless liquid.
    ii. It is miscible with water and organic solvents.
    iii. Acidic to litmus.
    iv. Reacts with iron to change its colour.
- *Storage*: It is stored in well closed, inert glass container below 30°C.

- *Incompatibility*: With base, alkalimetals metal, metal oxides, iron, oxidising agents.
- *Uses*
  i. As an acidifying agent.
  ii. In achlorhydria and hypochlorhydria.
  iii. In anaemia with iron therapy.

Q 4. Define antacids. Classify them. Give requirements for an ideal antacid. (S. 96, 99, 00, 01, 06, 07, 08, 09; W. 99, 01, 08)

Antacids

The substances which neutralize the abnormal or excessive acidity in stomach are called antacids.

Classification of Antacids

- *Water soluble (systemic) antacids*: Sodium bicarbonate.
- *Water insoluble (non-systemic) antacids*: Aluminium hydroxide gel, calcium carbonate, magnesium trisilicate, magnesium carbonate.

Requirements of an Ideal Antacid

- It should neutralize excessive acidity.
- It should not interfere with digestion.
- It should be stable.
- It should be nontoxic and nonirritant.
- It should not cause constipation.
- It should be cheap and easily available.
- It should be insoluble in water.
- It should not be absorbed through GIT.
- It should not evolve gas.
- It should not cause alkalosis.

Q 5. What are protectives and adsorbents? Give their actions and uses or write a note on protectives and adsorbents. (S. 98, 99, 00, 02, 03, 04, 05; W. 00, 01)

Protectives

These are the substances which protect the exposed surfaces from harmful stimuli, e.g. kaolin, bismuth carbonate.

Adsorbents

The substances which are used to adsorb the gases, toxins and bacteria are called adsorbents, e.g. kaolin, activated charcoal.

Gastrointestinal Agents 21

Mechanism of Action
- These substances are water insoluble and also insoluble in dilute HCl, alkali.
- These substances form a protective layer on innermost wall of GIT. Therefore, contact of bacterial toxins is prevented.
- Thus, stimulation of peristalsis by bacteria is prevented and they are used in diarrhoea.
- Adsorbents have a property to adsorb the bacterial toxins and also gases thus prevent attack of toxins on GIT.
- Frequent elimination of watery stools in diarrhoea can be prevented by protective adsorbents.

Examples

Bismuth subcarbonate, kaolin, activated charcoal.

Applications/Conditions in Which Protectives and Adsorbents are used
- They are useful in the treatment of diarrhoea.
- They are useful in poisoning cases to adsorb the poison.
- They prevent GIT irritation.
- They prevent entry of microbes in the body by forming protective layer, over the surfaces of the body.

Bismuth Compounds used as Protectives
- Bismuth subcarbonate.
- Bismuth subnitrate.
- Bismuth subgallate.
- Milk of bismuth.

Q 6. Write a note on "combination of antacid preparations". (S. 96, 97, 00, 03, 04, 06, 08; W. 96, 98, 99, 00, 01, 06, 08)

- There is no single antacid which is ideal. Therefore, combinations of antacids are used which reduce side effects and give more benefits.
- Antacid when given singly produces following complications:
  i. Sodium bicarbonate is quick acting but its side effect is systemic alkalosis.
  ii. Sodium-containing antacids may produce hypertension.
  iii. Magnesium compounds are contraindicated in patients with renal disorders.

22 Pharmaceutical Chemistry I

    iv. Calcium compounds are contraindicated in patients suffering from renal and cardiac disorders.
    v. Aluminium compounds should not be prescribed in patients having hypophosphatemia.
    vi. Aluminium and calcium compounds produce constipation.
    vii. Magnesium compounds may show laxative action.
- Combination of antacid is used because:
    i. Combination reduces constipation effect of antacids.
    ii. Combination reduces laxative action.
    iii. Some combinations produce specific action and are used for specific purpose.
    iv. Combination of drugs produces synergistic action.
    v. Combination also reduces the dose of drug required to produce action.
- Examples
    i. Calcium carbonate + aluminium hydroxide gel.
    ii. Calcium carbonate + magnesium trisilicate.
    iii. Magnesium trisilicate + aluminium hydroxide.

Q 7. Write in brief about (a) sodium bicarbonate, (b) bismuth subcarbonate, (c) kaolin.

(a) **Sodium Bicarbonate ($NaHCO_3$)** (S. 00, 01, 02, 03, 06, 08; W. 97, 99, 02, 04, 06)

- *Synonym*: Baking soda
- *Standard*: 99 to 100.5% w/w of $NaHCO_3$
- *Properties*
    i. White crystalline powder, odourless, saline taste.
    ii. Soluble in water and insoluble in alcohol.
    iii. Aqueous solution is alkaline.
    iv. On heating produces CO_2.
- *Storage*: Store in well closed containers.
- *Incompatibility*: With mercury salts and acid.
- *Uses*
    i. As an antacid.
    ii. As a carminative.
    iii. In treatment of crystaluria.
    iv. In treatment of systemic alkalosis.

v. In poisoning cases.
vi. In irrigation of eyes.
vii. In effervescent powders and bath soaps.

(b) Bismuth Subcarbonate (S. 07; W. 05)
- *Synonym*: Bismuth carbonate
- *Formula:* $[(BiO_2)\ CO_3]_2,\ H_2O$
- *Properties*
    i. White odourless, tasteless powder.
    ii. Insoluble in water and alcohol, dilute alkali.
    iii. Dissolves completely in HCl and in HNO_3.
    iv. Affected by light but stable in air.
- *Storage*: Store in well closed light resistant container.
- *Incompatibility*: With KI because it forms brown precipitation of bismuth tri-iodide.
- *Uses*
    i. As antidiarrhoeal.
    ii. Mild antiseptic and astringent.
    iii. In treatment of gastric and duodenal ulcers.
    iv. As a mild antacid.
    v. In treatment of colitis.
    vi. Used in cosmetics (lotions and face powder).

(c) Kaolin (S. 01, 02, 04, 05, 06, 07; W. 00, 01)
- *Synonym*: China clay
- *Properties*
    i. White odourless, tasteless powder.
    ii. Insoluble in water, dilute alkali and acids.
    iii. Available in two forms—heavy and light kaolin.
    iv. Impure forms of kaolin contain gritty particles.
- *Storage*: It is stored in well closed containers.
- *Incompatibility*: With vitamins, enzymes and alkaloids.
- *Uses*
    i. In treatment of dysentery and diarrhoea.
    ii. In treatment of alkaloidal poisoning.
    iii. In treatment of colitis.
    iv. In treatment of cholera.
    v. In food-poisoning cases.

vi. In dusting powders.
vii. In cosmetic preparations.
viii. As a main ingredient of kaolin poultice.

Q 8. Define purgatives, laxatives and cathartics. Classify purgatives with examples. (S. 97, 99, 00, 01, 05, 06, 07, 08, 09; W. 97, 99, 02, 03, 04, 05, 07)

Purgatives

The drugs which promote defaecation are called purgatives.

Laxatives

Mild purgatives are called laxatives.

Cathartics

Drastic purgatives are called cathartics.

Classification/Types of Laxatives

- *Stimulant/irritant purgatives*: Senna, phenolphthalein, castor oil.
- *Bulk purgatives*: Methyl cellulose, sodium carboxy methyl cellulose.
- *Emollient purgatives*: Liquid paraffin.
- *Saline cathartics*: Magnesium sulphate, sodium potassium tartrate.

Q 9. Write a note on "saline cathartics"/"saline purgatives". (S. 96, 98, 01, 09; W. 96, 97, 99, 00, 03, 07)

Saline Cathartics

Saline cathartics are the agents that quicken and increase evacuation from the bowels, e.g. magnesium sulphate, sodium potassium tartrate.

Mechanism of Action

- Saline cathartics increase osmotic pressure thereby secreting additional fluid in intestinal tract.
- This results in increase in bulk and stimulates peristalsis causing evacuation from the bowel.
- As saline cathartics increase the osmotic pressure and increase in peristalsis of GIT, they are used in the treatment of constipation.

Constipation

Constipation means hardening of stool which can be caused due to decreased peristaltic movements.

Gastrointestinal Agents 25

- Constipation may be due to intestinal injury, change in food intake, change in food type, change in environment, lack of exercise and due to consumption of medicinal agents.
- Thus, saline cathartics are mainly used in constipation.

Uses of Saline Cathartics

- To treat constipation.
- In hernia to avoid excessive straining.
- In haemorrhoids, boils and rectal disorders.
- To avoid rise in BP during defaecation.
- To remove intestinal contents before X-ray examination.

Q 10. Write a note on (a) magnesium sulphate, (b) sodium potassium tartrate.

(a) **Magnesium Sulphate** (S. 97, 98, 99, 00, 02, 03, 08; W. 97, 98, 02, 04, 05)

- *Formula*: $MgSO_4 \cdot 7H_2O$
- *Synonym*: Epsom salt.
- *Preparations*: It is prepared from magnesium carbonate and dil. H_2SO_4.

$$MgCO_3 + H_2SO_4 \rightarrow MgSO_4 + CO_2 + H_2O$$

- *Properties*
  i. Colourless crystals with cool and saline taste.
  ii. It is soluble in water.
  iii. It shows phenomenon of efflorescence in dry air.
  iv. It is odourless, very soluble in boiling water.
- *Storage*: It should be stored in well closed airtight containers in cool place.
- *Incompatibility*: With alkali, carbonate and bicarbonates, NaI, potassium tartrate.
- *Uses*
  i. As a saline purgative.
  ii. In treatment of heavy metal poisoning as antidote.
  iii. It is used for wet dressing.
  iv. In the treatment of boils.
  v. In hypertensive patients to avoid excessive straining.

(b) **Sodium Potassium Tartrate** (S. 99, 00, 03; W. 99, 00)

- *Synonym*: Rochelle's salt.

- *Properties*
  i. It is colourless, odourless crystalline powder.
  ii. It has a cooling saline taste.
  iii. It is soluble in water and insoluble in alcohol.
  iv. It shows phenomenon of efflorescence.
- *Storage*: Stored in tightly closed containers.
- *Incompatibility*: With acids, calcium and lead salts.
- *Uses*
  i. As a purgative.
  ii. As a stabilizer in cheese and meat products.
  iii. As ingredient of Fehling solution.
  iv. As ingredient of effervescent powders and bath soaps.

5

Topical Agents

Q 1. What are topical agents? Classify them with examples. (S. 96, 98, 00, 01, 02, 04, 05, 07; W. 01, 04, 08)

Topical Agents

The agents which are applied on the skin or mucus membrane for their local effects are called topical agents.

Classification

- On the basis of chemical origin
  - i *Organic topical agents*, e.g. zinc stearate, povidone iodine.
  - ii *Inorganic topical agents*, e.g. talc, zinc oxide, calamine.
- On the basis of action of drugs
  - i. *Protectives and adsorbents*, e.g. talc, zinc oxide.
  - ii. *Antimicrobial agents*, e.g. potassium permanganate, silver nitrate.
  - iii. *Astringents*, e.g. alum, zinc sulphate.
  - iv. *Miscellaneous compounds*, e.g. sulphur and its derivatives.

Q 2. Write a note on "topical protectives". (S. 96; W. 99, 00)

Topical Protectives

The substances which are used to protect the skin from external environment and applied on skin are called topical protectives.
- *Examples*: Talc, zinc oxide, calamine, titanium dioxide.
- They are available in the form of dusting powder, lotions, liniment, creams, ointment, etc.

Explanation

The substances having capacity to form a layer can protect the skin. These substances reduce mechanical friction, irritation, etc. These substances adsorb moisture and bacterial toxins and also protect skin from UV rays. These are insoluble in water and available in the form of powder. These are chemically and biologically inert and have good adsorption property, adequate flow property, sufficient covering capacity. These drugs are not adsorbed in circulatory system.

Applications
- To protect skin from sun-rays.
- To protect skin from bacterial toxins, dust and dirt particles.
- To protect skin from irritation and infections.
- To protect ulcers and wounds from external hazards.

Q 3. Write a note on "astringents". (S. 96, 01, 02, 07, 08; W. 96, 99, 00, 01, 02, 05, 06, 07)

Astringents

The substances which have a capacity to precipitate superficial proteins are called astringents, e.g. alum, zinc sulphate.

- *Dosage forms*: They are available in the form of dusting powders, mouthwashes, gargles, topical solutions, etc.

Explanation

Astringents are having less permeability and also very less penetration power. Therefore, when applied on skin, they are not affecting normal functioning of body cell.
- Astringents show following types of actions (Mechanism of action):
  i. *Styptic action*: Astringents precipitate surface proteins and blood proteins present at the site of wound. Therefore, diameter of blood capillaries is reduced. Due to constriction of capillaries and small blood vessels they show styptic action, i.e. to stop bleeding from small cuts.
  ii. *Anti-inflammatory action*: Astringents reduce blood supply coming towards the tissue and histamine secretion is also decreased. Thus, anti-inflammatory action is obtained.
  iii. *Antiperspirant action*: Astringents precipitate surface proteins thus decrease the diameter of sweat and sebaceous glands. Thus, perspiration is reduced, i.e. antiperspirant action.
  iv. *Antimicrobial action*: Astringents precipitate cell proteins of microbial cell, therefore, malfunctioning of microbial cell

Topical Agents 29

occurs. Further, microbial cell cannot get multiplied and thus antimicrobial action is achieved.

Applications/Uses of Astringents

- These are used as antimicrobial, anti-inflammatory, antiperspirants and styptic.
- In the treatment of wounds, ulcers, etc.
- In mouthwash and mouth freshener preparations.
- In toothpaste and tooth powder preparations.
- In dusting powders due to its antiperspirant action.

Q 4. Define and classify antimicrobial agents/anti-infective agents. (W. 96, 00)

Antimicrobial Agents

The substances which are used to kill microorganisms are called antimicrobial agents.

Classification of Antimicrobials

- *Antiseptics*: The substances which have a capacity to kill microbes and prevent the growth of microbes when applied on living material, e.g. hydrogen peroxide.
- *Disinfectants*: These are the substances having antimicrobial activity but used only for inanimate objects, e.g. cresol with soap solution.
- *Germicides*: Agents which kill the germs.
- *Fungicide*: Agents which kill the fungi.
- *Viricide*: Agents which kill the viruses.
- *Bacteriostatic*: Agents which stop the growth of bacteria.
- *Bacteriocidal*: Agents that kill the bacteria.
- *Preservatives*: These are the agents which prevent the contamination of products from microbes, e.g. methyl paraben.

Q 5. Give the mechanism of action of inorganic antimicrobial agents. (S. 00, 05, 06, 08; W. 96, 99, 01, 04, 08)

Antimicrobial agents may act by following mechanisms:
- *Oxidation*: Antimicrobial substances convert sulphidryl group to disulphide form. Therefore, disulphide group of proteins cannot work and thus kills microorganisms, e.g. hydrogen peroxide, $KMnO_4$.

- *Halogenation*: These substances add halogens to peptide linkage of microorganisms thus normal functioning of microbial cell gets disturbed, hence kills the microbes, e.g. iodine, povidone iodine, chlorinated lime.

- *Precipitation*: Many antimicrobial agents containing metal ions react with polar group of proteins and form a complex thus there is inactivation of protein (precipitation of proteins) and antimicrobial action is achieved, e.g. boric acid, borax, silver nitrate, mercuric compounds.

Q 6. Give the desirable ideal properties of antimicrobial agent used as topical anti-infective.

Ideal Properties of Antimicrobial Agents

- It should have rapid onset of action.
- It should have good therapeutic index.
- It should have sufficient antimicrobial action.
- It should be compatible with other ingredients.
- It should be economical and should be required in very less concentration.
- It should not have any type of toxicity.
- It should not damage host cell.
- It should have sustained action.
- It should have broad-spectrum action.
- It should have an adequate "lipid-water distribution coefficient".

Q 7. Write a note on "silicone polymers". (S. 99; W. 97, 99, 01, 02)

- Silicone polymers are inert protective substances occurring in liquid form and are generally known as silicone oils, e.g. simethicone, dimethicone.
- They are generally represented by formula

$$\left(CH_3-\underset{\underset{CH_3}{|}}{\overset{\overset{CH_3}{|}}{Si}}-C \left[-\underset{\underset{CH_3}{|}}{\overset{\overset{CH_3}{|}}{Si}}-O \right] -\underset{\underset{CH_3}{|}}{\overset{\overset{CH_3}{|}}{Si}}-CH_3 \right)$$

- *Properties*
  i. They are colourless, clear liquids.
  ii. They are water repellant (hydrophobic).

iii. They are stable to heat and affected by strong acids.
iv. They are soluble in light petroleum and in chloroform.
v. These are having —Si—O—Si— linkage.
- *Uses*
    i. Topical protective.
    ii. Gastric protective and antiflatulent.
    iii. As syringe lubricant.
    iv. Useful to protect bed sores.
    v. Simethicone is used as antispasmodic and mild sedative.
    vi. As a defoaming agent in antacids preparations.
    vii. Used in lotions, creams, ointments.

Q 8. Describe sulphur compounds used as topical agents. (W. 03, 08)

Sulphur compounds are:

(a) Sublimed sulphur, (b) Precipitated sulphur, (c) Selenium sulphide.

(a) Sublimed Sulphur (S. 00, 06, 07, 08; W. 01, 02, 08)

- *Synonym*: Flowers of sulphur.
- *Properties*
    i. It is fine, yellow crystalline powder.
    ii. Fine and slightly gritty having faint colour and taste.
    iii. Insoluble in water and alcohol.
    iv. It burns with a blue flame with production of sulphur dioxide.
- *Storage*: Store in a well closed container.
- *Uses*
    i. In the treatment of scabies (scabicide).
    ii. As a fungicide.
    iii. An ingredient of sulphur ointment.

(b) Precipitated Sulphur (S. 03, 06, 07, 08; W. 99, 08)

- *Synonym*: Milk of sulphur.
- *Properties*
    i. It is a pale greenish-yellowish soft powder.
    ii. It is odourless and tasteless.
    iii. Insoluble in water and alcohol.
    iv. It burns with a blue flame with production of sulphur dioxide.

- *Uses*
    i. As scabicide.
    ii. In seborrhoea, acne, pimples and psoriasis.
    iii. It also acts as keratolytic agents.

(c) Selenium Sulphide (S. 00, 06; W. 05, 08)
- *Formula*: SeS_2
- *Properties*
    i. It occurs as a bright orange powder with faint sulphide odour.
    ii. It is insoluble in water and alcohol.
    iii. It is tasteless.
    iv. It dissolves in HNO_3.
- *Uses*
    i. As antidandruff.
    ii. In seborrhoea.
    iii. In dermatitis.
    iv. For the treatment of scalp.
    v. Used in the form of shampoos.

Q 9. Write a note on (a) talc, (b) calamine, (c) titanium dioxide, (d) hydrogen peroxide, (e) potassium permanganate, (f) chlorinated lime.

(a) **Talc ($3 MgO \cdot 4 SiO_2 \cdot H_2O$) (S. 99, 06; W. 01, 05)**
- *Synonym*: French chalk
- *Properties*
    i. It is a fine, tasteless powder.
    ii. It is white in colour.
    iii. It is insoluble in water.
    iv. It has good flow property.
    v. It is physiologically and chemically inert.
- *Storage*: It is stored in a well closed container.
- *Uses*
    i. Topical protective.
    ii. As a dusting powder.
    iii. As a lubricating agent in tablet.
    iv. As a filter medium.
    v. As a distributing agent in aromatic waters.

(b) Calamine (ZnO + Fe₂O₃) (S. 96, 97, 98, 00; W. 98, 99, 01, 02, 03)
- *Properties*
    i. It is a pink, tasteless, odourless, fine powder.
    ii. It is physically and chemically inert.
    iii. It has good covering capacity.
    iv. It has good flow property.
    v. It is insoluble in water.
    vi. It has good absorption property.
    vii. It is soluble in dil. HCl.
- *Storage*: It is stored in a well closed container.
- *Uses*
    i. Topical protective.
    ii. Soothing agent.
    iii. As adsorbent.
    iv. Main component of make up preparation.

(c) Titanium Dioxide (TiO₂) (W. 05)
- *Properties*
    i. It is a white, odourless, tasteless powder, insoluble in water.
    ii. It is soluble in hot H₂SO₄ and HF.
    iii. It is amorphous.
- *Storage*: It is stored in a well closed container.
- *Incompatibility*: Incompatible with aluminium salts and alkali compounds.
- *Uses*
    i. Topical protective.
    ii. In cosmetic preparations and lotions.
    iii. In sunscreens, sun-burn creams and lotions.
    iv. In skin eruptions.
    v. In preparation of hard gelatin capsules.

(d) Hydrogen Peroxide (H₂O₂) (S. 97, 98, 99, 00, 05, 08, 09; W. 97, 00, 01, 02, 03, 06, 08)
- *Synonym*: Oxygenated water
- *Properties*
    i. It is colourless, odourless liquid with slight acidic taste.
    ii. Soluble in water, alcohol and ether.
    iii. It can be extracted with solvent ether from its aqueous solution.

34 Pharmaceutical Chemistry I

- *Incompatibility*: With reducing agents, oxidising agents, organic matter, heavy metals.
- *Stability storage*: It should be stored in light resistant containers with stoppers resistant to hydrogen peroxide. It should be stored in cool place.
  Label: The label should state whether or not the solution contains a stabilising agent.
- *Uses*
  i. Antiseptic, disinfectant
  ii. For cleaning of wounds
  iii. In mouthwash and gargles
  iv. Topical anti-infective
  v. Antimicrobial agent.

(e) **Potassium Permanganate ($KMnO_4$) (S. 97, 98, 99, 00, 05, 09; W. 97, 00, 01, 02, 06, 08)**

- *Properties*
  i. It is an odourless dark purple-coloured crystalline compound.
  ii. It has greenish-blue metallic lustre.
  iii. It has sweet astringent taste.
  iv. It is soluble in water.
  v. Its concentrated solutions are deep voilet.
  vi. When mixed with glycerin, it burns.
- *Incompatibility*: With iodides, reducing agents and organic substances.
- *Storage*: It should be stored in tightly closed container and avoid contact of organic matter. It should be handled with care.
- *Uses*
  i. As antimicrobial agent.
  ii. Powerful cleansing agent for wounds, ulcers.
  iii. In mouthwash and gargles.
  iv. As a deodorant.
  v. Antidote in barbiturate poisoning.
  vi. For gastric lavage treatment.
  vii. It leaves the stains on skin or tissues.

(f) **Chlorinated Lime (S. 01, 02, 03; W. 99, 02)**

- *Synonym*: Bleaching powder.

- *Properties*
    i. It is a dull white powder with odour of chloride.
    ii. It is slightly soluble in water and less soluble in alcohol.
    iii. On exposure, it absorbs moisture and forms chlorine gas.
- *Storage*: It should be stored in tightly closed container.
- *Incompatibility*: With oxidising agent, reducing agent.
- *Uses*
    i. Disinfectant.
    ii. Bleaching powder.
    iii. Bactericidal.
    iv. Used to disinfect wounds.
    v. In wet dressing.
    vi. As disinfectant in drinking water.

Q 10. Write a note on iodine and iodine preparations. (S. 96, 02, 03; W. 01)

Iodine preparations	Synonym
i. Aqueous iodine solution	
ii. Strong iodine solution	Lugol's solution
iii. Weak iodine solution	Tincture of iodine

- *Properties*: All are transparent brown-coloured liquids.
- *Uses*
    i. Aqueous solution of iodine used internally as a source of iodine
    ii. As a germicide and fungicide
    iii. Alcoholic solutions are antiseptics and disinfectants and applied on cuts and wounds.
    iv. Povidone Iodine: It is a complex of iodine and povidone.
- *Properties*
    i. It is yellowish-brown, amorphous powder.
    ii. It is hygroscopic.
    iii. Soluble in water and alcohol.
    iv. Aqueous solution is acidic and release iodine slowly.
- *Storage*: Store in an airtight, iodine resistant container.
- *Incompatibility*: With hydrogen peroxide.
- *Uses*
    i. Antiseptic.
    ii. 10% solution for cleaning of wounds.

iii. In gargles and mouthwashes.
iv. In vaginal infection.
v. In burns and cuts.

Q 11. Describe in brief the following compounds, (a) mild silver protein, (b) alum, (c) zinc sulphate, (d) povidone-iodine solution.

(a) **Mild Silver Protein (S. 98, 00, 02, 03, 05; W. 96, 97, 03)**
- *Properties*
    i. Dark brown or black shining granules.
    ii. Odourless and frequently hygroscopic.
    iii. Freely soluble in water.
    iv. It is affected by light.
- *Storage*: It should be stored in tightly closed glass container and protected from moisture and light.
- *Uses*
    i. Antibacterial.
    ii. To irrigate urethra and urinary bladder.
    iii. In respiratory tract infection.
    iv. In gonococcal infection.

(b) **Alum (S. 98, 00, 02, 05, 08; W. 96, 99, 01)**
- *Synonym*: Potash alum.
- *Properties*
    i. It is colourless, transparent crystalline mass.
    ii. It has sweetish and astringent taste.
    iii. It is very soluble in water and insoluble in alcohol.
- *Storage*: Store in a highly closed container.
- *Incompatibility*: Ca, lead and mercury salts.
- *Uses*
    i. As astringent.
    ii. Antiperspirant.
    iii. Local styptic.
    iv. In mouthwash and gargles, dusting powders.

(c) **Zinc Sulphate ($ZnSO_4 \cdot 7H_2O$) (S. 09; W. 03)**
- *Synonym*: White vitriol
- *Properties*
    i. Colourless, odourless transparent crystals with astringent taste.
    ii. Soluble in water, glycerin.

iii. Its aqueous solution is acidic to litmus.
  iv. It is efflorescent in dry air.
- *Storage*: Store in a tightly closed container.
- *Incompatibility*: With alkali, carbonate, borax.
- *Uses*
  i. As astringent.
  ii. Germicidal.
  iii. Styptic protective.
  iv. Emetic.
  v. In topical preparations.
  vi. In dermatological problems.

(d) **Povidone-iodine Solution (S. 97, 99, 00, 02, 08; W. 96, 99, 01, 03, 07)**
- *Properties*
  i. Povidone-iodine is a complex of iodine with povidone which is also a polymer, known as polyvinyl pyrrolidine (PVP).
  ii. The complex is a yellowish-brown amorphous powder and has characteristic odour.
  iii. Its aqueous solution is acidic to litmus.
  iv. It is soluble in water and in alcohol.
  v. The solution is transparent liquid having a reddish-brown colour and a pH not more than 6.0.
- *Action and uses*
  i. It has been used in gargles and mouthwashes.
  ii. For the management of burns and cuts.
  iii. Preparations are available to the skin and mucus membrane and for use as disinfectant.

6

Dental Products

Q 1. Write a note on dental products. OR Discuss various types of inorganic compounds used in dentistry and in dental products. (S. 96, 97, 99, 00, 01, 02, 07; W. 96, 97, 99, 00, 01, 02)

- Dental caries (tooth decay) is a disease of teeth which gives decalcification of tooth and bad odour of the mouth.
- To prevent dental caries and to maintain clean and healthy teeth, it is necessary to use dentifrices.
- Dentifrice may be toothpaste or tooth powders are used to clean dirty surface of teeth.
- Dental products are used in dentistry.
- Dental products are available in several dosage forms as toothpaste, tooth powders, silver polishes, oils, etc.
- Dental products contain:
  i. *Anticaries agents*: The agents which are used in the treatment of dental caries are called anticaries agents, e.g. sodium fluoride, stannous fluoride.
  ii. *Cleansing agents/abrasives*: These are the substances used to remove stain from the teeth, e.g. calcium phosphate, dicalcium phosphate, sodium phosphate.
  iii. *Polishing agents*: The substances which give whiteness to teeth by their abrasive action are called polishing agents, e.g. stannous fluoride, calcium carbonate.
  iv. *Desensitizing agents*: The substances which reduce the sensitivity of teeth to heat and cold are known as desensitizing agents, e.g. zinc chloride, strontium chloride.
  v. *Sweetening agent*: It gives sweet taste.
  vi. *Colouring agent*: It gives attractive colour to the preparation.
  vii. *Flavouring agent*: It provides pleasant flavour.

viii. *Humectant*: It prevents drying of toothpaste preparation, e.g. glycerin.

Q 2. Discuss the role of fluorides as anticaries. What is dental fluorosis? (S. 01, 07; W. 98, 99, 03, 08)

Anticaries

The substances which can prevent the formation of cavities in teeth are called anticaries agents.

Anticaries agents are fluorides, phosphates and ammoniated compounds.

Role of Fluorides

- Role of fluorides in preventing dental caries is well accepted.
- Administration of small quantity of fluorides in dental product may produce good results.
- Fluorides act as anticaries by two mechanisms:
    i. Fluorides decrease the solubility of enamel in lactic acid and also act against bacterial growth.
    Lactic acid is formed during the partial digestion of carbohydrates. This acid has ability to dissolve the enamel. Therefore, bacteria can localise on surface of teeth and thus cavities can be formed.
    ii. Fluorides act by inhibiting bacterial growth.
- Fluorides are having toxicity when they are taken in large quantity.
- When more quantity of fluoride is ingested, it is carried to bones and teeth and produces mottled enamel which is known as *dental fluorosis*. (S. 06; W. 06, 07)
- Fluorides are carcinogenic when deposited on teeth.
- When a fluoride-containing solution is taken (orally) internally it gets readily absorbed, transported and deposited in the bone or teeth and remainder is excreted by the kidneys.
- The deposited fluoride on the surface of teeth prevents the action of acids.

Sodium Fluoride: NaF (S. 98, 99, 00, 05, 08; W. 99, 02)
- *Properties*
    i. White odourless powder with slight bitter taste.
    ii. Soluble in water and insoluble in alcohol.
    iii. Reacts with ordinary glass.

- *Storage*: It should be stored in dark, pyrex bottles.
- *Uses*
    i. Dental products and anticaries agent.
    ii. 2% solution used topically.
    iii. It is used to treat abnormal development of teeth.

Q 3. Write a short note on (a) stannous fluoride, (b) dibasic calcium phosphate, (c) zinc chloride, (d) strontium chloride.

(a) Stannous Fluoride (S. 96, 00; W, 97, 02)

- *Formula*: SnF_2
- *Properties*
    i. White crystalline powder.
    ii. A bitter, salty taste.
    iii. Freely soluble in water, insoluble in alcohol.
    iv. It melts at 213°C.
- *Incompatibility*: It is incompatible with calcium pyrophosphate and with other calcium compounds.
- *Uses*
    i. Anticaries agent.
    ii. It is used in fluoride treatment of teeth.
    iii. A freshy prepared 8% solution of SnF_2 is applied to the cleaned dry teeth.

(b) Dibasic Calcium Phosphate (S. 98)

- *Synonym*: Calcium monohydrogen phosphate.
- *Formula*: $CaHPO_4$
- *Properties*
    i. White odourless powder with slight saline taste.
    ii. Insoluble in water and in alcohol.
    iii. Easily soluble in dil. HCl and HNO_3.
- *Storage*: It is stored in well-closed containers.
- *Uses*
    i. Electrolyte replenisher.
    ii. As a cleansing agent in toothpaste and powder.
    iii. As a source of calcium and phosphate.
    iv. Additive in tablet formulation.

(c) Zinc Chloride (S. 96, 98; W. 00, 01)
- *Synonym*: Buffer of zinc.
- *Formula*: $ZnCl_2$
- *Properties*
    i. White crystalline powder.
    ii. Odourless, tasteless.
    iii. Soluble in water, alcohol and glycerin.
    iv. It is deliquescent.
- *Storage*: It absorbs CO_2, therefore, should be stored in tightly closed containers.
- *Uses*
    i. Desensitizing agent.
    ii. Mild astringent, mild antiseptic.
    iii. Used in mouthwash and gargles.
    iv. Used in deodorant and talcum powders.

(d) Strontium Chloride (S. 96, 06; W. 00)
- *Formula*: $SrCl_2 \cdot 6 H_2O$
- *Properties*
    i. It occurs as colourless crystals or white granules.
    ii. Tasteless, odourless.
    iii. Soluble in water and alcohol.
    iv. It effloresces in dry air.
- *Storage*: It should be stored in well closed containers.
- *Uses*
    i. Desensitizing agent.
    ii. Used in toothpaste and tooth powder.

7

Inhalants

Q 1. Define inhalants. What is the role of oxygen and carbon dioxide in biological system? (S. 96, 98, 99, 00, 01, 06; W. 97, 99, 00, 01, 02)

Inhalants

The substances which are in vapour or gas form are inhaled through nose, are called inhalants, e.g. O_2, N_2O, CO_2.

Role of Oxygen (O_2)

- Oxygen is necessary in normal oxidative metabolism for the production of useful energy.
- This energy is used by the cell to synthesize ATP.
- After inhalation, O_2 enters into blood and combines with haemoglobin to form oxyhaemoglobin (HbO_2).
- This oxyhaemoglobin readily dissociates and releases oxygen in the medium of cell.
- Deficiency of oxygen in tissues is called hypoxia.
- Absence of oxygen in the tissues is called anoxia.
- When more oxygen is needed the condition is termed as asphyxia.
- For the treatment of hypoxia, anoxia and asphyxia, O_2 is needed.
- In the treatment of poisoning, O_2 is useful for maintenance of normal respiratory and circulatory functions.

Role of Carbon Dioxide (CO_2)

- CO_2 plays an important role in maintaining acid-base balance of the body.
- It is found in large quantity in plasma.
- It is readily absorbed and transported by blood both in cells and in plasma. It is also produced in the body during metabolic process.

Inhalants 43

- Carbonate buffer is physiological buffer which is useful in maintenance of acid–base balance of several body fluids.
- A large quantity of carbon dioxide produced is eliminated by lungs in expired air.
- Respiratory acidosis and respiratory alkalosis are the disorders produced due to imbalance of CO_2 level in the body.
- CO_2 stimulates respiratory centre and hence useful in treatment of carbon monoxide poisoning.

Q 2. Write a note on "oxygen". (S. 97, 02, 00, 08, 09; W. 00, 01, 06, 08)

Oxygen

- *Formula*: O_2
- *Standard*: Oxygen contains not less than 99% w/v of O_2.
- *Preparations*: By two methods:
  i. By electrolysis of water.
  ii. By fractionation of liquid air.
- *Properties*: By two methods:
  i. Colourless, odourless, tasteless gas.
  ii. It is a good oxidising agent.
  iii. It dissolves in about 32 volumes of water.
- *Storage and labelling* (W. 04)
  i. It is stored under the pressure in metallic cylinder which is painted by black and white colour. The body of the cylinder is painted by black and shoulder is painted with white colour.
  ii. Name and symbol of oxygen (O_2) is stenciled on cylinder and also on cylinder valve.
- *Actions and uses*
  i. In treatments of hypoxia, anoxia and asphyxia.
  ii. In carbon monoxide poisoning.
  iii. In cardiac arrest.
  iv. As a fuel in rocket technology.
  v. In the preparation of acetylene flame used for welding.

Q 3. Write a note on carbon dioxide. (S. 96, 97, 00, 08; W. 99, 07, 08)

Carbon Dioxide

- *Formula*: CO_2
- *Standard:* It contains not less than 99% w/v of CO_2.
- *Preparation*: Compounds containing carbon, e.g. coal, coke are burned in excess of O_2 to produce CO_2 $\qquad C + O_2 \rightarrow CO_2$

- *Properties*
    i. Colourless, odourless gas with faintly acidic taste.
    ii. Soluble in water and heavier than air.
- *Storage and labelling* (W. 04)
    i. It should be stored under pressure in a strong metallic cylinder.
    ii. The cylinder is painted grey colour at shoulder and remaining part may be of green or white colour.
- *Actions and uses*
    i. Respiratory stimulant.
    ii. In carbon monoxide poisoning.
    iii. In treatment of drug addiction.
    iv. Regulation of acid-base balance.
    v. Its salts are used in effervescent powders.
    vi. In preparation of soft drinks.
    vii. To prepare dry ice.
    viii. With O_2 for artificial respiration.

Q 4. Write a note on "nitrous oxide". (S. 02, 06; W. 00, 02)

Nitrous Oxide

- *Synonym*: 'Laughing gas'.
- *Formula*: N_2O
- *Standard*: It contains not less than 99% w/v of N_2O.
- *Preparation*: It is prepared by thermal decomposition of ammonium nitrate.

$$NH_4NO_3 \rightarrow 2H_2O + N_2O$$

- *Properties*
    i. It is colourless, odourless gas with slightly sweet taste.
    ii. It is soluble in water and alcohol.
- *Storage and labelling* (W. 04)
    i. It should be stored under pressure in a strong metallic cylinder below 37°C.
    ii. The cylinder is painted by blue colour.
    iii. The name and symbol of nitrous oxide (N_2O) are stenciled on cylinder and on the cylinder valve.
- *Actions and uses*
    i. In minor operations of boils (as anaesthetic).
    ii. In dentistry.
    iii. In mental patients (to calm).

8

Respiratory Stimulants

Q 1. Write a short note on respiratory stimulants. Explain ammonium carbonate/Discuss the role of ammonium compounds as respiratory stimulants. (S. 96, 00, 01, 02, 08; W. 96, 97, 99, 00, 01, 02, 03)

Respiratory Stimulants

The substances which increase the rate of respiration are called respiratory stimulants.

Classification

Respiratory stimulants are classified as:
- *Organic respiratory stimulants*: These are generally acting by central mechanism.
  - *Mechanism*: These stimulate the centre of respiration which is located in medulla oblongata, e.g. caffeine, theophylline, atropine.
- *Inorganic respiratory stimulants*: These are generally acting by reflux mechanism.
  - *Mechanism*: These substances either increase CO_2 concentration temporarily in blood or increase number of sensory stimuli through irritation, e.g. ammonium carbonate, aromatic spirit of ammonia.

Ammonium Carbonate

It is a mixture of ammonium bicarbonate and ammonium carbonate.
- *Formula*: $NH_4HCO_3 + NH_2CONH_4$.
- *Standard*: Not less than 30% of NH_3.
- *Properties*
  i. White crystalline powder.
  ii. Odour of ammonia.

iii. Volatile at room temperature.
iv. Decomposed by heat, hot water and acids.
v. Affected by light.
vi. Soluble in water and in alcohol.
vii. Its aqueous solution is alkaline to litmus.
viii. Also called "smelling salt".

- *Storage*: It should be stored in dark-coloured tightly closed container in a cool place away from light.
- *Uses*
  i. Respiratory stimulant.
  ii. Cough suppressant/expectorant.
  iii. Ingredient of aromatic spirit of ammonia.

9

Expectorants and Emetics

Q 1. Write a note on expectorants and emetics. (S. 96, 97, 99, 00, 01, 03; W. 96, 97, 98, 00, 01, 02, 05, 07)

(a) Expectorants

The drugs that remove sputum from the respiratory tract are known as expectorants.
- These drugs either increase the fluidity of sputum or increase the volume of fluids that are to be expelled from the respiratory tract by coughing.
- Expectorants are used orally to stimulate the flow of respiratory tract secretions.
- Expectorants are used in the treatment of respiratory disorders in which secretions are viscid or excessive, e.g. asthma.

Classification of Expectorants

According to mechanism of action expectorants are classified into two groups:

i. *Sedative type*: These act by irritating gastric mucosa thereby stimulating respiratory tract secretions, e.g. ammonium chloride, potassium iodide, syrup of ipecac, syrup of hydroiodic acid.

ii. *Stimulant type*: These drugs stimulate secretory cells of respiratory tract directly or indirectly and thus more fluid is produced in respiratory tract and sputum gets diluted, e.g. eucalyptus oil, lemon oil.

(b) Emetics

The drugs which produce vomiting are called emetics.
- These drugs remove fluid from respiratory tract and result in expulsion of stomach contents.

- Emetics are acting either by stimulating CTZ or by GIT irritation.
- Emetics are also classified into two groups:
  i. *Stimulant type*: These drugs stimulate CTZ in the medulla oblongata and induce vomiting, e.g. morpine, ergot alkaloids.
  ii. *Irritant type*: These are causing irritation of cells of GIT and by reflex mechanism vomiting is observed, e.g. antimony potassium tartrate, $CuSO_4$, NaCl.

Uses of Emetics

- These are given in combination with expectorants.
- These are used in treatment of poisoning to remove the poison from GIT.

Q 2. Write in brief about (a) ammonium chloride, (b) potassium iodide, (c) antimony potassium tartrate.

(a) **Ammonium Chloride (S. 00, 02, 04, 05, 06; W. 97, 02, 08)**

- *Formula*: NH_4Cl
- *Synonym*: Sal ammoniac, ammonium muriate.
- *Properties*
  i. White crystalline powder.
  ii. Colourless, odourless and has cooling, saline taste.
  iii. It is slightly hygroscopic.
  iv. It is more soluble in water but freely soluble in glycerine.
- *Incompatibility*: With alkalies, lead salts, warfarin.
- *Storage*: It is stored in tightly closed containers.
- *Actions and uses*
  i. As an expectorant
  ii. As an acidifying agent
  iii. To maintain physiological acid–base balance.
  iv. As a diuretic.

(b) **Potassium Iodide (W. 01, 03, 08)**

- *Formula*: KI
- *Properties*
  i. Colourless transparent crystals, slightly hygroscopic.
  ii. Saline bitter taste, soluble in water and glycerine.
  iii. Deliquescent, solution is alkaline.
- *Incompatibility*: With iron, copper, lead, mercury.

- *Storage*: In tightly closed light resistant container.
- *Uses*
    - i. As expectorant.
    - ii. As electrolyte replenisher.
    - iii. As a source of iodine.
    - iv. In treatment of hypothyroidism.
    - v. As stabiliser for iodine solution.

(c) **Antimony Potassium Tartrate (S. 01, 02; W. 97, 00, 02, 05)**
- *Formula*: $C_4H_4KO_7Sb$
- *Synonym*: "Tartar emetic", tartared antimony.
- *Properties*
    - i. Colourless, odourless crystals with saline taste.
    - ii. Soluble in water, insoluble in alcohol.
    - iii. It effloresces on exposure to air.
- *Storage*: It is stored in tightly closed containers.
- *Uses*
    - i. As expectorant, emetic.
    - ii. It acts as anti-schistosomal (schistosomiasis).
    - iii. IV injection of antimony potassium tartrate is useful in the treatment of kala azar.

10

Antidotes

Q 1. What are antidotes? Give the classification of antidotes. (S. 96, 97, 99, 00, 01, 02, 03, 05, 07, 08, 09; W. 96, 97, 00, 01, 02, 06, 07, 08)

Antidotes

The agents which are used to stop the action of poison are called antidotes.

Classification of Antidotes

On the basis of mechanism

- *Physiological antidote*: It changes the physiology so that effect of poison is countered/prevented, e.g. sodium nitrite, which converts haemoglobin into methemoglobin in order to bind cyanide.
- *Chemical antidote*: It reacts with poison and changes the chemical nature of poison and converts it into nonpoisonous compound, e.g. sodium thiosulphate, which causes conversion of toxic cyanide into nontoxic thiocyanide.
- *Mechanical antidote*: It prevents absorption of poison from GIT into the blood, e.g. activated charcoal, kaolin.
- *Universal antidote*: It is a combination of mechanical antidotes. It is useful when type of poison is not known or more than one poisons are consumed.
  Composition of universal antidote
  - Magnesium oxide   1 part
  - Tannic acid   1 part
  - Activated charcoal   2 parts

Q 2. Write a note on sodium nitrite. (S. 96, 00, 03, 08; W. 96, 98, 00, 01)

Sodium Nitrite

- *Formula*: $NaNO_2$.

- *Dose*: 10 to 15 ml of 2% solution by IV route.
- *Properties*
  i. White granular powder, saline taste.
  ii. It is deliquescent in air.
  iii. Freely soluble in water.
  iv. Solution alkaline to litmus.
- *Storage*: It should be stored in airtight containers.
- *Incompatibility*: With oxidising agents.
- *Uses*
  i. Antidote in cyanide poisoning.
  ii. An antioxidant.
  iii. Food preservative.
  iv. In *angina pectoris*.
  v. Antirusting for surgical instruments.
  vi. As smooth muscle relaxant.
  vii. As hypotensive drug.
  viii. As laboratory agent.

Q 3. Write a brief account on "cyanide poisoning". What is cyanide poisoning? Give the treatments of cyanide poisoning. (S. 96, 97, 99, 00, 01, 02, 03, 05, 09; W. 96, 97, 00, 01, 02, 07)

In cyanide poisoning, cyanide molecule reacts with ferric ion (Fe^{+++}) of cytochrome oxidase, which stops electron transfer and thereby stops cellular respiration.

Cyanide poisoning is very toxic, if it is not treated immediately.

Treatments of Cyanide Poisoning

- *Role of sodium nitrite*: Sodium nitrite reacts with haemoglobin to form methemoglobin. This methemoglobin reacts with serum cyanide and prevents entrance of cyanide in cell and thus cellular respiration is not affected.
- *Role of sodium thiosulphate*: Sodium thiosulphate reacts with cyanide ions and converts into sodium thiocyanate which is less toxic than cyanide. Sodium thiocyanate ion is excreted in urine.

$$Na_2S_2O_3 + CN^- \rightarrow SCN^- + Na_2SO_3$$

Along with sodium nitrite injection, sodium thiosulphate infusion (IV) is also given.
- *Role of activated charcoal and kaolin*: These are the mechanical antidotes useful to absorb the poisonous molecules present in the GIT, due to which blood concentration of poison is reduced.

11

Electrolytes

Q 1. Define electrolytes. Give types of electrolytes. (S. 04)

Electrolytes

The substances whose aqueous solutions conduct electricity are known as electrolytes.

Types of Electrolytes

- Major intracellular ions, e.g. K^+, Mg^{++}, HPO_4^{--}, $H_2PO_4^{-}$.
- Major extracellular ions, e.g. Na^+, Ca^{++}, Cl^-, bicarbonate.

Q 2. What is intracellular fluid (ICF) and extracellular fluid (ECF)? (S. 98, 03; W. 98, 00, 01, 02)

Intracellular Fluid (ICF)

It means fluid present inside the cell, e.g. cytoplasm.

Extracellular Fluid (ECF)/Interstitial Fluid

It means fluid present between the cells, e.g. tissue fluid.

The Plasma (Vascular Fluid)

It means the fluid present within the blood vascular system.
- *Anionic electrolytes*, e.g. HCO_3^-, Cl^-, SO_4^{--}, HPO_4^-.
- *Cationic electrolytes*, e.g. K^+, Ca^{++}, Na^{++}, Mg^{++}.

Q 3. Write a note on "oral rehydration therapy/salts/ORT/ORS". (S. 99, 00, 01, 02, 06, 08, 09; W. 96, 98, 99, 00, 01, 03, 04, 06)

- These are orally administered electrolyte solutions used to supply water and electrolytes needed to the patients.
- A large number of formulations of oral rehydration preparations are available in the market.

- These preparations contain glucose, sodium chloride, potassium chloride, sodium bicarbonate. These may contain flavouring agents.
- These are dry powdered preparations and are mixed with water and taken orally.
- ORS are made available at free of cost by government of India.
- It is available at PHC generally at free of cost.
- ORS available in market are electrol powder, paediatric powder.
- ORS contains

NaCl	3.5 gm
KCl	1.5 gm
Sodium citrate	2.9 gm
Glucose	20 gm

- This mixture is added in 1 litre of water and then taken by oral route.
- It is the first aid remedy in condition of dysentery, diarrhoea, prolonged fever, vomiting, etc.

Q 4. Give a brief account of "electrolyte combination therapy". (S. 96, 97, 00)

Electrolyte Combination Therapy

Electrolytes are combined together in a definite quantity for the specific purpose, which is called electrolyte combination therapy.

- When patient is unable to take normal diet before or after surgery the electrolyte combination therapy is used. For this purpose, infusion containing dextrose and NaCl is used.
- As per need of the patient combinations of electrolytes are prepared and given to the patients.
- After surgery nutrients and electrolytes are used for physiological acid-base balance.
- In dysentery, diarrhoea, prolonged fever, vomiting, the loss of electrolytes is observed which is supplied by electrolyte solutions.
- Various electrolyte combinations available in the market are divided into two groups:
    i. Fluid maintenance group.
    ii. Electrolyte replacement group.

i. *Fluid Maintenance Group*

- All the fluid maintenance of electrolyte infusions contains at least 5% dextrose, which helps to reduce starvation.

- It is given after surgery or to the patients who do not take food orally.
- These solutions of electrolytes are administered intravenously which provide the normal requirement of water and electrolytes.
- The electrolytes used in combination with dextrose are Na^+, K^+, Ca^{++}, Cl^-, Mg^{++}, phosphate.

ii. *Electrolytes Replacement Group/Replacement Therapy*
- This electrolyte replacement therapy is required when there is an excessive loss of water and electrolytes in diarrhoea, vomiting, sweating and prolonged fever, etc.
- Electrolyte replacement group contains infusions which are used as replacement fluids. These are of two types:
    i. A solution for rapid initial replacement.
    ii. A solution for subsequent replacement.
- Initially for rapid replacement the Na^+ ions are more and K^+ ions are less and reverse in next.
- Formula for electrolyte combination therapy
    i. General use:

Sodium chloride	1 gm	
Potassium chloride	1.5 gm	for 1 litre of solution
Sodium bicarbonate	1.5 gm	
Anhydrous glucose	30.4 gm	
Glucose	40 gm	

    ii. WHO and UNICEF recommended formula

NaCl	3.5 gm	
KCl	1.5 gm	for 1 litre of solution
$NaHCO_3$	2.5 gm	
Anhydrous glucose	20 gm	
Glucose	22 gm	

- Electrolyte replacement therapy includes:
    i. Infusions.
    ii. Powders for oral solutions.
- Electrolyte infusions available are:
    i. Sodium lactate injection IP, BP.
    ii. Compound sodium chloride injection IP (Ringer's solution).
    iii. Compound sodium lactate injection IP (Ringer's lactate solution).

Q 5. Write the monograph of sodium chloride.

Sodium Chloride (S. 99, 02, 07, 09; W. 97, 00, 01, 02, 07)
- *Formula*: NaCl.
- *Standard*: It contains not less than 99.5% of NaCl.
- *Properties*
  i. It is a white crystalline powder.
  ii. It is odourless, saline taste (salt).
  iii. Freely soluble in water.
  iv. It is hygroscopic.
- *Storage*: Store in well closed container.
- *Uses*
  i. As a source of sodium and chloride.
  ii. As electrolyte replenisher.
  iii. In bromide and iodide poisoning.
  iv. In foods.
  v. In kidney failure.
  vi. Along with diuretics.
  vii. To maintain isotonicity of solutions.
  viii. Topically to wounds and body cavities for irrigation.
- *Official preparations/formulations of NaCl*
  i. Sodium chloride and mannitol injection IP, USP.
  ii. Sodium chloride hypertonic solution IP, BP.
  iii. Compound NaCl injection IP, BP, USP.
  iv. Normal saline solution IP, BP.
  v. Dextrose and normal saline solution IP, BP.
  vi. Sodium chloride eye lotion BP.
  vii. Sodium chloride tablet IP.
  viii. Compound NaCl and dextrose solution BP.
  ix. Compound sodium chloride and dextrose powder BP.
  x. Bacteriostatic sodium chloride injection USP.
  xi. Ringer's injection USP.
  xii. Mannitol and sodium chloride injection.
  xiii. Fructose and sodium chloride injection, NF.
  xiv. Lactated Ringer's injection.
- *Category*: Systemic alkalizer, electrolyte replenisher.
- Deficiency of sodium chloride known as "salt hunger".

56 Pharmaceutical Chemistry I

Q 6. Write the monograph of potassium chloride. (S. 97, 04; W. 97, 99)

Potassium Chloride (KCl)
- *Standard*: It contains not less than 99.5% of KCl.
- *Properties*
  i. Colourless crystals or white crystalline powder.
  ii. Odourless with saline taste.
  iii. Its aqueous solution is neutral to litmus.
  iv. Freely soluble in water.
- *Storage*: Store in well closed container.
- *Uses*
  i. As electrolyte replenisher.
  ii. As ingredient of Ringer's solution.
  iii. In treatment of paralysis.
  iv. In *myasthenia gravis*.
  v. Antidote in digitalis poisoning.
- *Official compounds/formulations of potassium chloride*
  i. Potassium chloride oral solution USP.
  ii. Potassium chloride injection IP, USP.
  iii. Potassium chloride and sodium chloride IV infusion BP.
  iv. Potassium chloride tab USP.
  v. Potassium chloride and dextrose IV infusion BP.
  vi. Lactated Ringer's injection USP.
  vii. Ringer's solution IP, BP, USP.
  viii. Compound sodium chloride injection IP.
  ix. Lactated Ringer's injection USP.
  x. Lactated potassium saline injection NF.

Q 7. Write a note on (a) metabolic acidosis, (b) metabolic alkalosis, (c) respiratory acidosis, (d) respiratory alkalosis.

(a) Metabolic Acidosis (S. 00, 01, 02, 06, 07; W. 99, 00, 01, 02, 03, 07, 08)

It means a disturbed acid–base balance of the body and physiological fluids become acidic in nature. In this case, pH is decreased below 7.35.
- *Causes*
  i. Failure to excrete metabolic acids by kidney.
  ii. Due to diarrhoea, vomiting or diabetes mellitus.
  iii. Excess absorption of metabolic acids.
  iv. Loss of base from the body.

- *Treatment*: Sodium acetate, sodium citrate, potassium citrate, potassium acetate.

(b) **Metabolic Alkalosis (S. 00, 01, 02, 06, 07; W. 99, 00, 01, 02, 03, 07, 08)**
It means a disturbed acid–base balance of the body and physiological fluids become more alkaline in nature. In this case, pH is increased more than 7.45.
- *Causes*
    i. Excessive ingestion of alkaline drugs.
    ii. Use of diuretics.
- *Treatment*: Ammonium chloride and its injection.

(c) **Respiratory Acidosis**
It is the state in which carbon dioxide is retained in the body due to reduced ventilation.
- *Causes*
    i. Due to mechanical/muscular impairment.
    ii. Disease of lung due to CNS depression.

(d) **Respiratory Alkalosis**
It is the state in which excess of carbon dioxide is lost from the body and it is due to hyperventilation.
- *Causes*
    i. Due to emotional factors.
    ii. Fever.
    iii. Salicylate poisoning.

Q 8. Give the meaning of hypokalemia, hyperkalemia, hyponatremia, hypernatremia.

- *Hypokalemia*: It means loss of potassium from the body.
- *Hyperkalemia*: It means excess of potassium in the body.
- *Hyponatremia*: It means loss of sodium from the body.
- *Hypernatremia*: It means excess of sodium in the body.

Q 9. Explain how physiological acid–base balance of the body is maintained? (S. 99, 02, 06, 08; W. 96, 00, 01, 02, 08)

- All the body fluids have definite composition of enzymes, ions, proteins, etc.
- Generally majority of metabolic reactions are happened at pH range 7.34–7.42.

- The pH of body fluid is maintained by following mechanisms:
  i. *Buffer system*: Carbonate buffer systems and phosphate buffer systems maintain acid–base balance. This system is mainly found in kidney and cells.
  ii. *Protein buffer system*: Proteins are composed of amino acids which dissociate and give H^+ and thus participate in buffering of the body fluids. Haemoglobin is the most effective buffer.
  iii. *Respiratory mechanism*: The important pH control is through the control of "respiratory centre". When this centre is stimulated, it alters the rate of breathing.

  The removal of CO_2 from the body fluids leads to the changes in pH of blood carbonic acid.
  iv. *Renal mechanism*: Kidney helps to maintain normal pH by elimination of some ions through urine. Kidney has an ability to form ammonia which reacts with acid formed during protein metabolism and thus pH of urine is acidic.

  If any one of these mechanisms is not functioning properly, metabolic/respiratory acidosis or alkalosis may occur.

12

Official Compounds of Iodine, Iron and Calcium

Q 1. Give the official compounds, incompatibility, storage, action and uses of iron compounds. (S. 98, 02, 04, 08, 09; W. 00, 06)

Official Compounds of Iron

The following iron compounds are official in IP 1985:
i. Ferrous fumarate.
ii. Ferrous gluconate.
iii. Ferrous sulphate.
iv. Dried ferrous sulphate.
v. Iron and ammonium citrate.
vi. Iron sorbitol injection BP
vii. Ferrous succinate BP } Official in BP.
viii. Iron dextran injection BP

- *Incompatibility*: Iron compounds are incompatible with mineral acids, alkali, alkali-carbonates, tannates.
- *Storage of iron salts;* They undergo oxidation thus are stored in airtight containers in cool and dark place.
- *Actions and uses of iron compounds*
    i. In iron-deficiency anaemia.
    ii. In haemorrhage condition.
    iii. As haematinics
        - *Anaemia*: It means decrease in percentage of haemoglobin or RBCs in the blood.
        - *Haematinics*: The substances which increase the number of RBCs in the blood are known as haematinics.

Q 2. Give the official compounds, incompatibility, storage and uses of iodine compounds. (S. 96, 97, 98, 05, 07, 08, 09; W. 98, 01, 08)

Official Compounds of Iodine

The following are official compounds of iodine:
  i. Sodium iodide.
  ii. Potassium iodide.

- *Incompatibility*: With oxidising agents, reducing agents.
- *Storage*: Sodium and potassium iodides are deliquescent in moist air and are oxidised giving yellowish or brown colour due to liberation of iodine.

  Thus iodine compounds are preserved in a well-closed container and kept in dry place.

- *Uses*
  i. In disorders of thyroid gland (goitre).
  ii. As fibrinolytic agent in syphilis and leprosy.
  iii. In fungal infections.
  iv. Potassium iodide is used in cough mixtures as expectorants.
  v. Useful in asthma and chronic bronchitis.

- *Deficiency disorders of iodide*: Deficiency of thyroid hormones causes hypothyroidism. It involves:
  i. *Cretinism*: It involves mental retardation and dwarfism.
  ii. *Goitre*: It involves enlargement of thyroid gland and swelling of neck.

Q 3. Mention the official compounds, incompatibility, storage, uses of calcium compounds. (W. 98)

Official Compounds of Calcium

Following are the official compounds of calcium in IP 85:
  i. Calcium carbonate.
  ii. Calcium chloride.
  iii. Calcium hydroxide.
  iv. Calcium gluconate.
  v. Calcium lactate.
  vi. Calcium amino salicylate.

vii. Calcium pentothenate.
viii. Tribasic calcium phosphate.
ix. Calcium levulinate.
x. Dibasic calcium phosphate.
- *Incompatibility*: With phosphate, sulphate, oxidising agents.
- *Storage*: Stored in airtight, light resistant container.
- *Uses*
  i. As a source of calcium.
  ii. Calcium replenisher in lactation and pregnancy.
  iii. In treatment of tetany, rickets, osteomalacia, hypocalcemia.
  iv. In combination with vitamin D in treatment of osteomalacia.
- *Biological importance of calcium ions*
  i. Essential for normal function of ANS.
  ii. For normal cardiac function.
  iii. For coagulation of blood.
  iv. For growth of bones and teeth.
  v. For muscle contraction.

13

Radioactivity

Q 1. Define radioactivity. Give types of radioactivity. (S. 99, 02; W. 96, 99, 01, 02, 06)

Radioactivity

Radioactivity is a spontaneous and continuous emission of α, β, γ radiations from the substances.

Types of Radioactivity

- *Natural radioactivity*: It is observed spontaneously and continuously without any external efforts, e.g. radium^{226}, iodine^{131}.
- *Artificial radioactivity*: It is called induced radioactivity and produced by bombardment of high velocity particles on an element, e.g. bombardment of α-particles on nitrogen converts it into radioactive oxygen.

Q 2. Define the units of measurement of radioactivity.

- *Curie*: It is the quantity of any radioactive substance undergoing the same number of disintegrations in unit time as that of 1 gm of radium.
- *Rad*: It is defined as the quantity of radiation which releases or absorbs 100 erg/gm of specified medium.
- *Roentgen*: It is the unit of measurement of ionising effect of radiation by measuring damaging effect on biological matter.

Q 3. Define the terms—Isotopes, isobars, isotones, nuclide, nuclear isomers. (S. 96, 98, 01; W. 98)

- *Isotopes*: The species which have different atomic mass number but the same atomic number are called isotopes, e.g.

$$^{206}_{82}Pb, \ ^{207}_{82}Pb \ ^{208}_{82}Pb$$

- *Isobars*: The atoms of different elements having different atomic numbers and same atomic mass numbers are called isobars, e.g. $_6^{14}C$ & $_7^{14}N$
- *Isotones*: Atomic species having same number of neutrons but different mass numbers are called isotones.
- *Nuclide*: Nuclide is a species of atom characterized by the constitution of the nucleus, in particular by the number of protons and neutrons in the nucleus.
- *Nuclear isomers*: Atoms of the same elements having same atomic number and same atomic mass number but differ in radioactive properties are called nuclear isomers.

Q 4. Distinguish between isotopes and isobars.

Isotopes	*Isobars*
i. They have the same atomic number but different atomic mass number.	i. They have the same atomic masses but different atomic numbers.
ii. They have the same number of protons, but different number of neutrons.	ii. They have different number of protons, as well as neutrons.
iii. They have similar physical and chemical properties.	iii. They have different physical and chemical properties.
iv. They occupy the same place in the periodic table.	iv. They occupy different places in the periodic table.

Q 5. Give/compare the properties of α, β, γ radiations. (S. 96, 98, 02, 06, 08; W. 96, 98, 99, 01, 02, 06)

α-particles	*β-particles*	*γ-particles*
i. When α-particle is emitted, the atomic number decreases by 2 and mass number decreases by 4.	• When β-particle is emitted, the atomic number is increased by 1 and mass number is not changed.	• When γ-radiations are emitted, there is no change in atomic or mass number.
ii. α-particles are positively charged particles.	• They are positively charged but negatively charged	• They do not have charge but have energy.

Contd.

α-particles	β-particles	γ-particles
	particles are most common.	
iii. Penetration power is low.	• Penetration power is more than α-particles.	• Penetration power is more than α and β-particles.
iv. Ionisation power is very high.	• Ionisation power is less than α-particles	• Ionisation power is very less.
v. They have low speed.	• They have more speed than α-particles.	• They have equal speed to that of light.
vi. They are affected by strong magnetic and electric fields.	• They are affected by strong magnetic and electric fields.	• They are not affected by strong magnetic and electric fields.
vii. No application in pharmacy.	• No application in pharmacy.	• Useful in sterilization.
viii. It is identical with helium nucleus $_2He^4$.	• It is represented as $_{-1}^{0}e$	• It is represented as $_{0}^{1}n$

Q 6. What precautions are to be taken in handling and storage of radioactive materials? (S. 96, 97, 03, 06; W. 96, 99, 00, 01, 06, 07)

- Radioactive substances should never be touched with hand, but handled with forceps.
- Activities like smoking, drinking, eating should be avoided in the area where radioactive substances are kept.
- Sufficient protective clothing should be used during handling of radioactive substances.
- Area where the radioactive materials are kept should be tested regularly for the presence of fluorescence.
- There should be proper disposal of radioactive materials.
- Radioactive materials may be kept in a suitable, labelled container.
- They should be kept in remote area.
- All surfaces of the containers should be smooth, nonporous, non-wetting, and heat resistant.

- Fluorescence should be removable.
- The wall finishes should be hard and smooth and should not easily get contaminated.
- The amount of wood material should be minimum.
- The benches, cupboards should be made up of plastics.
- There should be minimum movement of workers.
- Workers should wear protective clothes while entering the area where radioactive materials are stored.

Q 7. Enlist various methods/devices used for measurement of radiations/radioactivity. (S. 96,98, 99, 00, 01, 02, 09; W. 96, 00, 02, 07, 08)

- Ionisation chamber.
- Proportional counters.
- GM counters (Geiger-Müller counter).
- Scintillation counters.
- Semiconductor detectors.
- Photographic plate method.

Q 8. Give the construction and working of GM counters (Geiger-Müller counters). (S. 07, 08, 09; W. 07, 08)

Geiger-Müller Counters

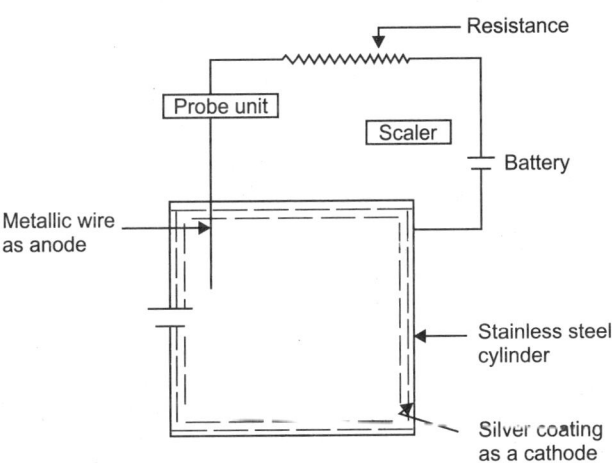

Construction and Working

- It consists of stainless steel or glass cylinder coated with silver on the inner side which acts as a cathode.

- A fine metal wire is mounted coaxially inside the cylinder which acts as an anode.
- The cylinder is filled with argon gas.
- Radiations enter through the window.
- Due to radiations, argon gas is ionized.
- A high voltage (800–1300 V) is maintained between the electrodes.
- Due to ionization of argon gas, positively charged ions are attracted towards cathode and negatively charged ions are attracted towards anode.
- The passage of these ions through the tube constitutes flow of current.
- Each particle of radiation causes a brief flow or pulse of current which is recorded by a device known as "scaler".
- Scaler shows total number of pulses and results are analysed.

Q 9. What are radiopaque contrast media? Give ideal requirements of radiopaque substance. Explain $BaSO_4$. (S. 96, 97, 99, 04, 05; W. 96, 98, 00, 01, 02, 03, 05, 06)

Radiopaque Contrast Media (X-ray Contrast Media)

The substances which have a capacity to prevent passage of X-rays and hence are opaque on X-ray examination are called radiopaque substances. The medium which gives this type of phenomenon is called radiopaque contrast medium.

Radiopaque substances are administered by oral route and very rarely by IV route.

Ideal Properties Requirements of Radiopaque Substance

- It should prevent the passage of X-rays.
- It should have an adequate radiopacity.
- It should be stable.
- It should have high solubility.
- It should be nontoxic.
- It should be chemically and physiologically inert.
- It should have a capacity to accumulate at desired site for desired time.
- It should be easily excreted from the body.

Barium Sulphate (S. 96, 98, 99, 02; W. 00, 01, 02, 05)

- *Formula*: $BaSO_4$
- *Synonym*: Barium meal, shadow meal.

Preparation

It is prepared by precipitation of barium ions from cold and dilute solution of barium salt with dil. H_2SO_4. The ppt. is washed and dried.

$$BaCl_2 + H_2SO_4 \longrightarrow BaSO_4 + 2\ HCl$$

Properties
- It is a fine, white, odourless, tasteless and bulky powder.
- It is insoluble in water.
- It is not absorbed from GIT.
- It is soluble in concentrated H_2SO_4.

Dose
200 to 400 gm orally.

Actions and Uses
- Used for X-ray examinations of alimentary canal.
- Orally or by enema for examination of colon.
- Used for the preparation of barium sulphate compound powder.

Q 10. Explain "biological effects of radiation". (S. 04, 08, 09)

The effects of radiation on living matter are called biological effects.

Biological Effects of Radiations

(a) Ionization and Excitation
- Radiations cause abnormal chemical effects such as inactivation of essential enzymes, coagulation of proteins.
- Ionization of nucleic acid like DNA and RNA damages the cell.

(b) Skin Damage

When skin is exposed to radiations, it may cause:
- Reddening of skin.
- Blackening of skin.
- Loss of hair.
- Dryness of skin.
- Burning of skin.

(c) Somatic Effects

Effects of radiations on blood cells are called somatic effects.
    These are caused due to excessive exposure to radiation. These include:

- Anaemia
- Leukaemia
- Cancer
  i. Somatic effects are observed after many years from exposure.
  ii. The cancer is observed generally after 20 years from exposure.

(d) Genetic Effects

Genetic effects are:
- Damage to chromosomes.
- Change in frequency of gene mutation.
- Due to genetic effects, abnormal effects are observed in future generation.

Q 11. What are applications/uses of radioisotopes/radiopharmaceuticals? (S. 96, 97, 98, 99, 00, 01, 06, 08; W. 96, 97, 98, 99, 00, 02, 04)

Radioisotopes are used:
- In medicine for therapeutic and diagnostic purpose.
- In research for study of metabolic processes.
- For synthesis of several compounds.

Some important radioisotopes are:
- Calcium (^{44}Ca and ^{45}Ca): It is used to study bone structure and in treatment of bone cancer.
- Cobalt (^{60}Co): It is used for sterilisation of surgical dressings.
- Cyanocobalamin (^{57}Co): It is used in the diagnosis of pernicious anaemia.
- Gold (^{198}Au): In the treatment of cancer.
- Iodine: To study thyroid uptake.
- Hydrogen (^{2}H, ^{1}H): It is used to determine total body water.
- Oxygen (^{17}O, ^{18}O): Used in study of photosynthesis.
- Sodium (^{22}Na, ^{24}Na): For the estimation of extracellular fluid.
- Iron (^{55}Fe, ^{59}Fe): To measure lifespan of RBCs.
- Carbon (^{14}C): For metabolism of carbohydrates and fats.

Q 12. Define half-life of radioelement. (S. 04, 06, W. 03, 04)

Half-life

It is the time in which the amount of radioactive substance is decreased to ½ of its original.

$$t\tfrac{1}{2} = \frac{0.693}{\lambda} \quad \lambda = \text{Decay constant}$$

14

Quality Control of Drugs and Pharmaceuticals

Q 1. Define quality control. Give functions and importance of quality. (S. 96, 99, 00, 02, 03, 05, 07; W. 99, 01, 02, 03, 05, 06, 07)

Quality Control

It is the day-to-day process of controlling quality of every incoming material till the finished product quality.

Functions of Quality Control

- Analysis of raw materials.
- Analysis of packaging materials.
- Analysis of in-process products.
- Analysis of final dosage forms.
- Analysis of batch products (periodic analysis).
- Recording the results of analysis in a standard format.

Importance of Quality Control

- To avoid toxic and unwanted effects of impurities.
- To avoid technical difficulties during manufacturing.
- To maintain safety and effectiveness of products.
- To maintain product with adequate physical and chemical stability.
- To ensure quality drugs for consumption to the patients.
- To maintain purity of product and thus protect public health.
- To help in maintenance of quality of product with better utilization of labours and machines.
- It helps in adjustment and setting of machineries.
- It helps in product development and in research with control over wastes and scraps.
- It helps in decreasing the cost of manufacturing so that cost of final product may be decreased.

Q 2. Define quality assurance. Give its functions. (W. 03, 05, 06)

Quality Assurance

It is the department which includes a total quality control, government regulations, company standards and development of standard operating procedures of analysis.

Functions

- Development of standard operating procedures and supply to every department of the company.
- It has a responsibility of "total quality of the products".
- It gives guidelines during adjustment and setting of the machineries.
- It helps to maintain quality of products with better utilisation of labours and machines.
- It helps in product development and research.

Q. 3. What are different methods used for quality control in pharmacy? (S. 99, 00; W. 98)

Quality control is to analyse a drug for quality and quantity. Following are various methods used for quality control.

Quality Control Methods

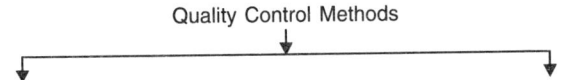

A. Qualitative analysis
  i. By colour, odour, solubility
  ii. Identification tests
  iii. Boiling point, melting point

B. Quantitative analysis
  (Estimation of % of drug, i.e. assay)
  i. Chemical assay methods
    a. Volumetric analysis:
      – Acidimetry and alkalimetry
      – Redox titrations
      – Precipitation titrations
      – Complexometric titrations
    b. Gravimetric analysis
      – Estimation of weight
  ii. Photometric methods
  iii. Electrochemical methods
  iv. Biological assay methods

Quality Control of Drugs and Pharmaceuticals 71

Q 4. Write in short about "significant figures". (S. 96, 98, 04, 07; W. 98, 00)

Significant Figures

Significant figures can be defined as the number of digits necessary to express the results of measurement consistent with the measured precision.

- It should be clear that zeros are used to denote the significant part of measurement.
- Thus, zeros within a number like 25.05 and 1350 are significant as they express the exact quantity while in the quantity 0.0035 kg, the zeros are not significant figures.

Q 5. Write a note on "errors in analysis". (S. 97, 98; W. 97)

Error

Error is the difference between measured value and true value.

- Though the measurements are made by different methods of quality control, systematically and carefully but there is some degree of error.

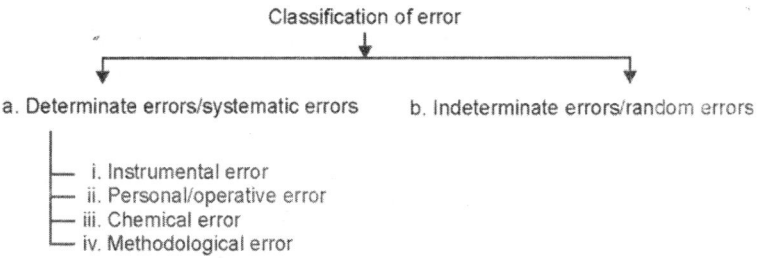

a. Determinate errors/systematic errors
    i. Instrumental error
    ii. Personal/operative error
    iii. Chemical error
    iv. Methodological error

b. Indeterminate errors/random errors

a. *Determinate errors/systematic errors*: These types of errors are determinable and can be either avoided or corrected.
   i. *Instrumental error*: It is caused by use of faulty equipment.
   ii. *Personal error*: It is the error made by person doing analysis.
   iii. *Chemical error*: This error is due to impurities in chemicals.
   iv. *Methodological error*: It arises due to faulty method used for analysis, e.g. incomplete reaction, incomplete heating.

b. *Indeterminate errors/random errors*: These errors are also called accidental errors. These errors are fluctuating and do not have a definite value and are difficult to locate. They arise due to unknown and uncertain measurement or may be due to differences in judgement and skill of analyst.

Hence, elimination of these errors is impossible to the analyst.

Q 6. Define impurity. Discuss various sources of impurities in pharmaceutical substances. (S. 96, 98, 99, 06, 07, 08, 09; W. 97, 98, 99, 00, 01, 02, 03, 04, 05, 06, 08)

Impurity

Impurity is an undesirable matter which may or may not be toxic but present in the pharmaceutical substances.

Sources of Impurities

- *Raw material used in manufacture*: If raw material contains an impurity, then this impurity gets incorporated into the final product.

  Impurities like lead, arsenic, etc. are present in the raw materials and hence found in substances as impurities, e.g. if copper foils are contaminated with arsenic, the final product $CuSO_4$ may contain arsenic impurity.

- *Reagents used in manufacturing process*: If reagents contain impurity, it is transferred to the final product, e.g. calcium carbonate is prepared by using calcium chloride and sodium carbonate. Thus it may contain impurity of sodium carbonate or calcium chloride.

- *The process used in manufacturing*: There are a number of chemicals which are manufactured from different raw materials by different methods or processes. Due to this some impurities get incorporated into the materials during manufacturing process.

  Tap water is generally used in various manufacturing processes. Tap water contains chlorides, calcium, magnesium as impurities thus gets incorporated in the products.

- *Material of plant*: Equipment and vessels used in manufacturing process are made of metals like copper, iron, aluminium, zinc but these metals are introduced as impurities by the solvent action of raw materials. Nowadays, these metals are replaced by stainless steel.

- *Intermediate products*: Incomplete reactions produce unwanted intermediate products which may be the impurity in the final products.

- *Adulteration/accidental substitution*: The cheap substances are added in pure substances as a substitute and, therefore, added substances act as an impurity in pure substance, e.g. sodium bromide is an impurity in potassium bromide as the sodium salt is cheaper.

Quality Control of Drugs and Pharmaceuticals 73

- *Inadequate storage/defective storage*
  i. Many chemical substances undergo changes due to careless storage, thus may develop impurity in it.
  ii. Stored products may become contaminated with dust, the bodies of insects and even animals and insect excreta.
  iii. Many substances when exposed to light, air and moisture, may change the colour, properties and shelf life of products, e.g.
     - Due to careless storage, ferrous sulphate is slowly converted into insoluble ferrous oxide by air and moisture.
     - Surgical solution of chlorinated soda deteriorates upon exposure to light and heat. Hence, it should be stored in well closed amber-coloured bottles in cool place.
     - Chloroform decomposes in presence of light and air and forms a phosgene gas which is toxic. So it should be stored in well closed amber-coloured bottle.
     - Bismuth carbonate is blackened on long exposure to sunlight.
- *Manufacturing hazards*: Impurity may get incorporated at various stages of manufacturing.
  i. *Particulate contamination*: It involves the pieces of plastic, threads in the product and also come from improperly cleaned equipment and also due to wear and tear of equipment.
  ii. *Process error*: It involves incomplete reactions during processing.
  iii. *Cross-contamination*: Handling of powders, granules and tablets may produce considerable air-borne dust. This air-borne dust may lead to cross-contamination of other products.
  iv. *Microbial contamination*: Liquids or creams may be contaminated due to bacteria and fungi from atmosphere.
  v. *Packing errors*: The products of similar appearance such as tablet of same size, colour and shape may be packed in the similar containers and can cause danger due to mislabelling.

Q 7. What are different types of Impurities commonly occurring in pharmaceuticals? (W. 99)

- *Toxic impurity*: If impurity is present above the prescribed limit and produces toxic effect on the body, it is called toxic impurity, e.g. lead, arsenic impurities.

74 Pharmaceutical Chemistry I

- *Harmless impurity*: Some impurities are harmless but if present above the prescribed limit, they lower active strength of substances, e.g. impurities of sodium salts in potassium salts.
- *Impurity affecting storage property*: For example, presence of small amount of moisture in the drug may reduce flow property and affect the storage.
- *Impurity causing technical difficulties*: Impurities cause many technical problems during manufacturing, e.g. picking and sticking defects may occur in tablet manufacturing.
- Impurities affecting taste, odour and appearance of the product.
- Impurities even when present in traces, may show a cumulative toxic effect after certain period.
- Impurity which lowers the shelf life of the substances.

Q 8. Discuss the effects of impurities. (S. 96; W. 01)

Effects of Impurities

- Impurities may produce toxic effect if present above certain limits.
- Impurities, even in small quantity, may show cumulative toxic effect after a certain period.
- Impurities may reduce active strength of the substance.
- Impurities may change physical and chemical properties of the substance and thus making it medically useless.
- Impurities may cause technical difficulties in the formulations.
- Impurities may produce incompatibility with other substances.
- Impurities may lower the shelf life of the substance.
- Impurities may affect and change the colour, odour, taste and appearance and make the substance unhygienic.

Q 9. What do you mean by 'test for purity'? Mention various tests for purity of the substance. (W. 00, 05)

Tests for Purity

These are the tests used for detecting impurities in the substances.
- Following are the tests for purity:
    i. Colour and odour.
    ii. Physical constants (MP, BP).
    iii. Humidity.
    iv. Insoluble constituents.
    v. Acidity and alkalinity.
    vi. Organic impurities.

vii. Ash value.
viii. Loss on drying (LOD) ⎫
ix. Loss on ignition (LOI) ⎬ (S. 04)
x. Anions and cations.

Q 10. Define the term "limit tests". Explain BSR.

Limit Tests (S. 96, 99, 04, 09; W. 08)

These are qualitative tests used to identify the small amounts of impurities present in the substances.

BSR (Barium Sulphate Reagent) (S. 96, 99; W. 08)

It is used in limit tests for sulphate IP 85.
- *Composition of BSR*
  i. $BaCl_2$ solution.
  ii. Sulphate-free alcohol.
  iii. Potassium sulphate solution.
- *Uses of ingredients*
  i. $BaCl_2$ reacts with impurity to form $BaSO_4$.
  ii. Alcohol prevents supersaturation.
  iii. Potassium sulphate increases the sensitivity of test.

Q 11. Describe the limit test for chloride IP. (S. 96, 98, 99, 01, 04, 05, 09; W. 96, 97, 00, 01, 02, 03, 05, 07)

Principle/Concept

Chloride impurity reacts with silver nitrate to form a white precipitate of silver chloride in the presence of dilute HNO_3. It is observed as opalescence.

Reaction

$$Cl^- + AgNO_3 \xrightarrow{\text{dilute } HNO_3} AgCl \downarrow + NO_3^-$$

Silver nitrate → Silver chloride precipitation

Note
- Purified water is used for dilution and it is free from dissolved gas and impurities.
- Standard solution is prepared as it gives maximum permissible limit for comparison.
- Dilute HNO_3 is used as it avoids the reaction of acidic radicals other than chloride with that of $AgNO_3$.

- The opalescence is directly proportional to amount of chloride impurity present in the substance.
- If test substance is coloured (KMnO$_4$), then first it is decolourised and then followed for limit test.

Procedure

Limit test for chloride IP 66	
Test solution	*Standard solution*
i. Weight of substance as per monograph. ii. 1 ml of dilute HNO$_3$. iii. Dilute up to 50 ml with water. iv. Add 1 ml of 5% AgNO$_3$ solution.	i. 1 ml of 0.01 N HCl solution. ii. 1 ml of dilute HNO$_3$. iii. Dilute with water up to 50 ml. iv. Add 1 ml of 5% AgNO$_3$ solution.
Limit test for chloride IP 85	
Test solution	*Standard solution*
i. Weight of substance as per monograph. ii. Add 10 ml of dilute HNO$_3$. iii. Add water up to 50 ml. iv. Add 1 ml of 1% AgNO$_3$ solution.	i. 1 ml of 0.0585 w/v of NaCl solution. ii. Add 10 ml of dilute HNO$_3$. iii. Add water up to 50 ml. iv. Add 1 ml of 1% AgNO$_3$ solution.
Limit test for chloride IP 96	
IP 96 prescribes use of 1 ml of 0.1 M AgNO$_3$ solution. The chloride impurity is generally 25 parts per million. Standard chloride solution is taken 10 ml for the preparation of standard solution.	

Stir both the solutions and keep it aside for 10 minutes.

Remarks

If opalescence produced in test solution is less than standard solution, substance passes the limit test for chloride IP.

Q 12. Describe the limit test for sulphate IP. (S. 96, 00, 02, 04, 05, 07; W. 97, 99, 02, 06, 07, 08)

Principle/Concept

Sulphate impurity reacts with barium chloride in the presence of dilute HCl to form white precipitation of barium sulphate. It is observed in the form of turbidity.

Reaction

$$SO_4^{--} + BaCl_2 \xrightarrow{\text{dilute HCl}} BaSO_4 \downarrow + 2Cl^-$$

Barium chloride → Barium sulphate precipitation

Note

- Purified water is used for dilution and it is free from dissolved gas and impurities.
- Standard solution is prepared as it gives maximum permissible limit for comparison.
- Dilute HCl is used as it avoids the reaction of acidic radicals other than sulphate with that of $BaCl_2$.
- Barium sulphate reagent: It is used according to IP 85. It contains $BaCl_2$, K_2SO_4 and alcohol. Barium chloride reacts with sulphate impurity. Alcohol prevents supersaturation. Potassium sulphate increases rate of reaction and sensitivity.

Procedure

Limit test for sulphate IP 66	
Test solution	*Standard solution*
i. Weight of substance as per monograph.	i. 2.5 ml of 0.01N H_2SO_4.
ii. 1 ml of dilute HCl.	ii. 1 ml of dilute HCl.
iii. Add water up to 50 ml.	iii. Add water up to 50 ml.
iv. Add 1 ml of $BaCl_2$ solution.	iv. Add 1 ml of $BaCl_2$ solution.
Limit test for sulphate IP 85	
Test solution	*Standard solution*
i. Weight of substance as per monograph.	i. 1 ml of 0.1089% w/v of K_2SO_4.
ii. Add 2 ml of dilute HCl.	ii. Add 2 ml of dilute HCl.
iii. Add water up to 45 ml.	iii. Add water up to 45 ml.
iv. Add 5 ml of BSR.	iv. Add 5 ml of BSR.
Limit test for sulphate IP 96	
It prescribes ethanolic sulphate standard solution which gives 10 ppm sulphate impurity and also use of 25% w/v barium chloride solution.	

Stir well both the solutions and keep it aside for 5 minutes.

Remarks

If turbidity produced in test solution is less than standard solution, sample comply with the limit test for sulphate IP.

Q 13. Describe the limit test for iron IP. (S. 96, 99, 00, 01, 03, 05, 06, 08, 09; W. 96, 00, 01, 02, 05, 06, 08)

Principle/Concept

Iron impurity reacts with thioglycolic acid in the presence of dil. ammoniacal alkaline medium to form purple-coloured ferric thioglycate.

Reaction

$$Fe^{++} + 2 \begin{array}{c} CH_2-SH \\ | \\ COOH \end{array} \xrightarrow{Ammonia} \left(\begin{array}{c} CH_2-SH \\ | \\ COO \end{array} \right)_2^{Fe} + 2H^+$$

Thioglycolic acid → Ferric thioglycate (purple-coloured)

Note

- Purified water is used for dilution purpose and it is free from dissolved gases and impurities.
- Standard solution is prepared as it gives maximum permissible limit for comparison.
- Ammoniacal alkaline medium is necessary for reaction of thioglycolic acid with iron impurity.
- Citric acid prevents precipitation of iron with ammonia.
- Thioglycolic acid is used because it reacts with ferrous form of iron and converts it into ferric form. Thus, it forms purple colour.

Procedure

Limit test for iron IP 66

Test solution	Standard solution
i. Weight of substance as per monograph.	i. 2 ml of standard iron solution (0.173 gm of ferric ammonium sulphate + 1.5 ml of HCl).
ii. Add 40 ml of water.	ii. Add 40 ml of water.
iii. Add 2 ml of citric acid (20%).	iii. Add 2 ml of citric acid.
iv. Add ammonia to adjust alkaline pH.	iv. Add ammonia to adjust alkaline pH.
v. Adjust volume up to 50 ml with water.	v. Adjust volume up to 50 ml with water.

Contd.

Limit test for iron IP 85	
Test solution	*Standard solution*
i. Weight of substance as per monograph.	i. 2 ml of standard iron solution (0.1726 gm of ferric ammonium sulphate + 10 ml of 0.1 N H_2SO_4).
ii. Add 40 ml of water.	ii. Add 40 ml of water.
iii. Add 2 ml of citric acid.	iii. Add 2 ml of citric acid.
iv. Add ammonia to adjust alkaline pH.	iv. Add ammonia to adjust alkaline pH.
v. Adjust volume up to 50 ml with water.	v. Adjust volume up to 50 ml with water.

Stir well and keep aside for 5 minutes and observe.

Remarks

If purple colour obtained in test solution is less than standard solution, sample passes limit test for iron IP.

Q 14. Describe the limit test for heavy metals IP. (S. 96, 03, 04; W. 97, 04, 07, 08)

Principle/Concept

Heavy metal impurity reacts with hydrogen sulphide/sodium sulphide in presence of acidic/alkaline medium respectively to form brown precipitation of metal sulphide.

Reaction

i. $M + H_2S \longrightarrow MS + 2H^+$

ii. $M + NaS \longrightarrow MS + 2Na^{++}$

(Metal sulphides) (brown precipitations)

Note

- Purified water is used for dilution purpose and it is free from dissolved gases and impurities.
- Standard solution is prepared as it gives maximum permissible limit for comparison.
- H_2S and Na_2S solutions are the reactants and require acidic/alkaline media for their reactions respectively.

- Acidic medium is adjusted by ammonia or acetic acid while alkaline medium is adjusted by NaOH.
- IP 66 does not have limit test for heavy metals.

Procedure

Method 'A'

Limit test for heavy metal IP 85	
Test solution	*Standard solution*
i. As per monograph 25 ml solution prepared.	i. Take 2 ml standard lead solution and dilute it up to 25 ml.
ii. Add dilute acetic acid/ ammonia to adjust the pH between 3 and 4.	ii. Add dilute acetic acid/ ammonia to adjust the pH between 3 and 4.
iii. Add water up to 35 ml.	iii. Add water up to 35 ml.
iv. Add 10 ml of H_2S solution.	iv. Add 10 ml of H_2S solution.
v. Dilute it up to 50 ml with water.	v. Dilute it up to 50 ml with water.

Stir well and keep aside for 5 minutes. Observe and compare the brown colour produced.

Remarks

If brown colour obtained in test solution is less than standard solution, sample passes the limit test for heavy metal IP 85.

Q 15. Describe the limit test for arsenic. (S. 96, 97, 98, 99, 01, 06, 07, 08, 09; W. 96, 98, 00, 01, 02, 04, 05, 06, 07)

Principle/Concept

Arsenic impurity is converted into arsine gas which further reacts with mercuric chloride paper to form yellow stain of mercuric arsenide.

Reactions

i. Arsenic is converted into arsenic acid.

$$As \longrightarrow H_3AsO_4$$

ii. Arsenic acid is converted into arsenous acid.

$$H_3AsO_4 \longrightarrow H_3AsO_3$$

iii. Arsenous acid is converted into arsine gas.

$$H_3AsO_3 + 6[H] \longrightarrow AsH_3 \uparrow + 3H_2O$$
$$\text{(Arsine gas)}$$

iv. Arsine gas is converted into mercuric arsenide.

$$2AsH_3 + HgCl_2 \longrightarrow Hg\begin{matrix}\diagup AsH_2 \\ \diagdown AsH_2\end{matrix} + 2HCl$$

Mercuric arsenide (yellow stain)

Note
- Purified water is used for dilution purpose and it is free from dissolved gases and impurities.
- Standard solution is prepared as it gives maximum permissible limit for comparison.
- Lead acetate cotton plug is used to avoid the interaction of hydrogen sulphide gas with mercuric chloride.
- Stannated zinc is used for slow and steady evolution of nascent hydrogen.
- Time required for the preparation is more therefore, this test should be observed after 40 minutes.
- All reagents should be having AST grade (free from arsenic).

Procedure

Limit test for sulphate IP 85	
Test	Standard
i. Substance as per monograph.	i. 0.2 to 1 ml standard arsenic solution.
ii. Add 1 gm of KI.	ii. Add 1 gm of KI.
iii. Add 10 gm of stannated zinc	iii. Add 10 gm of stannated zinc.

Shake the bottles and keep aside for 40 minutes.

Remarks

If yellow stain obtained in test mercuric chloride paper is less than standard stain, sample passes limit test for arsenic IP 85.

Q 16. Describe apparatus used for limit test for arsenic. Explain Guitzeit test apparatus. (S. 99, 01, 05, 06, 08, 09; W. 99, 00, 01, 03, 06, 07, 08)

Guitzeit Test Apparatus

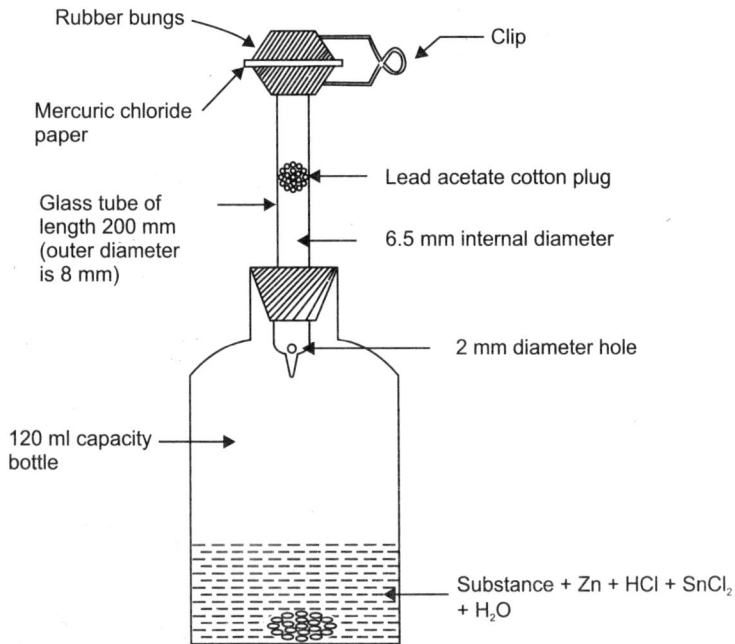

Construction

- It consists of a wide-mouthed glass bottle of capacity 120 ml.
- Glass tube of 200 mm length is passed in it through the rubber bungs.
- Glass tube is constricted at lower end.
- It has a 2 mm hole.
- The end of the tube should be above the liquid.
- Mercuric chloride paper is sandwitched between two rubber bungs and fixed by clip.
- Lead acetate cotton plug is inserted into the glass tube before operation.

Board Question Papers
(From Summer 1996 to Summer 2017)

Summer Examination 1996
D Pharm First Year
Pharmaceutical Chemistry I

Q 1. Attempt any *five* of the following:
- a. What are limit tests? Explain reactions and principle involved in limit test of chlorides.
- b. Write a note on antacid combinations.
- c. How do manufacturing hazards affect the purity of pharmaceuticals?
- d. What are inhalants? Give the properties and uses of nitrous oxide or carbon dioxide.
- e. Give the formula, uses, properties and incompatibilities of ferrous sulphate or calcium gluconate.
- f. Give one official identification test of (any *four*):
  - i. Calcium
  - ii. Iodides
  - iii. Chlorides
  - iv. Sodium
  - v. Lactate
  - vi Citrate
- g. What is quality control? Discuss its importance in pharmaceutical industry.

Q 2. Attempt any *two* of the following:
- a. Write a note on (any *two*):
  - i. Measurement of radioactivity.
  - ii. Handling and storage of radioactive materials.
  - iii. Applications of radioisotopes.
- b. i. What do you know about antidotes? How are they classified? Explain the role of sodium nitrite in cyanide poisoning.
  - ii. What are expectorants? Name any two inorganic expectorants. Write an account of any one of them.

c. Draw and label the arsenic testing apparatus IP. Discuss the principle behind the limit test for arsenic. Give reactions.

Q 3. Attempt any *two* of the following:
- a. i. Give the properties, storage conditions and uses of potassium permanganate or hydrogen peroxide solutions.
  - ii. Discuss limit test for sulphate. Give the significance of barium sulphate reagent.
- b. i. What are desensitizing agents? Give properties, formula and uses of chlorides of zinc or strontium.
  - ii. What are radiopaque contrast media? Give properties and uses of $BaSO_4$.
- c. Make a list of major intra- and extracellular electrolytes categorising them as anionic and cationic. Give a brief account of electrolyte combination therapy.

Q 4. Attempt any *two* of the following:
- a. i. Discuss in brief various sources of impurities in pharmaceuticals.
  - ii. Explain the principle behind the limit test for iron.
- b. Give formula, properties and uses of (any *two*):
  - i. Stannous fluoride
  - ii. Sodium metaphosphate
  - iii. Calcium carbonate
- c. i. What are cathartics? Write a note on saline cathartics.
  - ii. Write a brief account of ammonium carbonate as a respiratory stimulant.

Q 5. Attempt any *two* of the following:
- a. i. Compare the properties of α, β, γ radiations.
  - ii. Write a note on biological effects of radiations.
- b. i. What are topical agents? Classify them giving examples.
  - ii. What do you know about antioxidants? What are the criteria for selection of inorganic oxidants? Give properties of sodium metabisulphite.
- c. Write a note on (any *two*):
  - i. Standard buffers
  - ii. Limit test for heavy metals
  - iii. Significant figures

Q 6. Attempt any *two* of the following:
- a. What are antacids? How are they classified? Give requirements of an ideal antacid. Discuss any one antacid agent.

b. Define and give one example (any *six*):
  i. Acid
  ii. Base
  iii. Acidifying agent
  iv. Astringent
  v. Antimicrobial agent
  vi. Anticaries agent
  vii. Radioisotope
c. i. What are topical protectives? Give important properties and uses of calamine or talc.
  ii. Give the properties of iodine and discuss the official preparations of iodine.

Winter Examination 1996
D Pharm First Year
Pharmaceutical Chemistry I

Q 1. Answer any *five* of the following:
a. Define acids and bases. Give properties, uses and storage conditions of boric acid.
b. Write basis for selection of antioxidants. Give properties and uses of (any *two*) of the following:
  i. Nitrogen
  ii. Sodium thiosulphate
  iii. Sodium metabisulphite
c. Name two compounds used to treat hyperacidity. Explain GIT protective and astringents with examples.
d. Give properties and uses of the following compounds (any *two*):
  i. Talc
  ii. Povidone-iodine
  iii. Alum
  iv. Mild silver protein
e. Define the terms:
  i. Dentifrices
  ii. Contrast media
  iii. Buffers
  iv. Saline cathartics
f. Match the following pairs:

A	B
i. Silver nitrate	1. Painted blue
ii. Oxygen cylinder	2. Filter aid
iii. Nitrogen cylinder	3. Foils or collapsible tubes
iv. Titanium dioxide	4. Treatment of cancer
v. Kieselguhr	5. Relief of dental hypersensitivity
vi. Aluminum metal	6. Chemical antidotes
vii. Colloidal gold injection	7. Caustic astringent
viii. Strontium chloride	8. Source of impurities

86 Pharmaceutical Chemistry I

    ix. Sodium thiosulphate
    x. Cross-contamination
    9. Painted black
    10. Whitening agent
    11. Mechanical antidote

Q 2. Answer any *three* of the following:
- a. Explain inorganic inhalants. Write uses, storage and precautions during handling of inhalants.
- b. Define the terms:
  - i. Respiratory stimulants
  - ii. Emetics
  - iii. Expectorant

  Name at least two examples of each.
- c. Define antidotes. Name the universal antidote. How are they classified? Write properties and action of sodium nitrate.
- d. Name the compounds used in the treatment of metabolic acidosis and alkalosis, comment on their properties and storage conditions.

Q 3. Answer any *three* of the following:
- a. Explain combination antacid preparations and give their advantages.
- b. Write medicinal uses of following (any *four*):
  - i. Borax
  - ii. Chlorinated lime
  - iii. Epsom salt
  - iv. Sodium chloride
  - v. Zinc oxide
- c. Name the compound used in (any *four*) treatment of the following:
  - i. Peptic ulcer
  - ii. Sub burn
  - iii. Polycythemia-vera
  - iv. Hyperthyroidism
  - v. Achlorhydria
  - vi. Eczema
  - vii. Fungal infection
- d. What are hematinics? Describe the compounds used and their official preparations.

Q 4. Answer any *three* of the following:
- a. Explain physiological acid–base balance and mention at least six electrolytes used in the acid–base imbalance.
- b. Draw outline diagrams and explain working of the instruments used for radioactivity measurements. Or
Give any four applications, with handling, storage and labelling of radiopharmaceuticals.
- c. Explain the principle involved in the limit test for arsenic with suitable reactions.
- d. Write identification test for the following cations (any *two*):
  - i. Calcium
  - ii. Ferrous
  - iii. Bicarbonate

Q 5. Answer any *three* of the following:
a. Give official procedure of the limit test for chloride and iron.
b. Explain principle involved in the limit test for iron with reactions.
c. Explain oral rehydration therapy. Give composition of ORS recommended by UNICEF. Explain the role of calcium and sodium in body.
d. Define radioactivity. Give any three properties of alpha, beta and gamma rays. Explain in brief biological effect of radiations.

Q 6. Answer any *three* of the following:
a. Write medicinal uses of the following:
   i. Magnesium trisilicate
   ii. Zinc chloride
   iii. H_2O_2
   iv. Calamine
b. Give the properties and uses of kaolin. Name the official preparations.
c. Give synonyms and formula:
   i. Bleaching powder   v. Talc
   ii. Sodium hydroxide   vi. Borax
   iii. Magnesium oxide   vii. Precipitated sulphur
   iv. Magnesium sulphate   viii. Alum
d. Define antiseptic and disinfectants. Explain mechanism of action of inorganic antimicrobial agent.

Summer Examination 1997
D Pharm First Year
Pharmaceutical Chemistry I

Q 1. Solve any *five* of the following:
a. Explain buffers, their role in pharmaceutical preparations with examples. Mention acetate or phthalate buffer.
b. Give properties, uses, storage conditions and chemical incompatibility of following (any *one*):
   i. Boric acid   ii. Calcium hydroxide
c. Give the importance of various gastrointestinal agents. Name the inorganic compounds and their uses.
d. Classify laxatives and give advantages and disadvantages of magnesium sulphate as a saline cathartic.
e. Discuss the properties and uses of sodium bicarbonate and comment on the incompatibilities produced.

f. Match the following pairs:
- i. Hydrochloric acid
- ii. Thioglycolic acid
- iii. Alum
- iv. Talc
- v. Geiger-Müller counter
- vi. Curie (ci)
- vii. Mercury (Hg)
- viii. Milk of sulphur

1. Haemostatic
2. Radioactivity
3. Mild antiseptic, parasiticide
4. Unit of radioactivity
5. Mobile liquid
6. Protective dusting powder
7. Achlorhydria
8. Reagent for iron impurity

Q 2. Solve any *three* of the following:
a. Give an account of antioxidants commonly used. What is the basis for their choice?
b. Explain the effect of heat on following:
   - i. Boric acid
   - ii. Sodium thiosulfate
   - iii. Potassium permanganate
   - iv. Yellow mercuric oxide
c. Give the physical, chemical properties, IP standard, storage and uses of ammonia solution or hydrogen peroxide.
d. Give uses and incompatibilities produced by the following compounds (any *four*):
   - i. Sodium nitrite
   - ii. Iodine
   - iii. Potassium chloride
   - iv. Gold (Au^{198})
   - v. Potassium permanganate

Q 3. Answer any *three* of the following:
a. Explain any *one* of the following:
   - i. Silver nitrate as antimicrobial
   - ii. Antidotes
b. Give official preparations and their IP standards for sodium chloride and iodine.
c. Name the inorganic compounds valuable in the treatment of cough. Write their properties.
d. Describe the role of oxygen and CO_2 Or magnesium and calcium in the body.

Q 4. Answer any *three* of the following:
a. Explain types of errors in quantitative analysis. Discuss in process quality control.
b. Define radiopharmaceuticals. Give their applications, handling, storage and labelling.
c. Give chemical properties, uses, storage and handling of sodium hydroxide Or Discuss hematinic compound.

Q 5. Solve any *three* of the following:
a. Explain electrolytes and combination of electrolytes. What is maintenance and replacement therapy of electrolyte?
b. Explain with example (any *one*):
   i. Emetics
   ii. Sampling of pharmaceuticals
   iii. Combination of antacids.
c. What is calamine and povidone iodine? Give their applications.
d. Define buffers. Discuss the advantages and disadvantages of important buffer used in pharmacy Or Discuss in short about dental products.

Q 6. Solve any *three* of the following:
a. Fill in the blanks:
   i. Hydrolysis of oils and fats by NaOH is known as _____.
   ii. Zinc oxide forms cement-like mass when mixed with strong solution of _____.
   iii. Iodophosphorous are complex of iodine with _____.
   iv. Hypoxaemia is corrected by giving _____.
b. Give official procedure of limit test for arsenic Or lead impurity as per IP 1985.
c. Write chemical formula, uses, synonyms of following (any *four*):
   i. Talc
   ii. Calcium carbonate
   iii. Kaolin
   iv. Magnesium sulfates
   v. Borax
   vi. Ammonium carbonates
d. Name the inorganic compound used in following (any *eight*):
   i. Warts
   ii. Ulcers
   iii. Gangrenes
   iv. Corns
   v. Decolorising agents
   vi. Filter aids
   vii. Preservatives
   viii. Eye infection
   ix. Poisoning due to insecticides
   x. Filter aids
   xi. Dandruffs

Winter Examination 1997
D Pharm First Year
Pharmaceutical Chemistry I

Q 1. Answer any *five* of the following:
a. How is lead incorporated in pharmaceutical compounds? How will you perform limit test? Explain.

b. Discuss in short:
   i. Errors in quantitative analysis.
   ii. Sampling during analysis of various formulation and importance of quality control.
c. Discuss biological effects of radiation. Write application of radiopharmaceuticals.
d. Write uses and official preparations of:
   i. Sodium phosphate P^{32}
   ii. Ammonium chloride
   iii. Sodium lactate
e. Write definitions of:
   i. Buffers
   ii. Antioxidants and preservatives
   iii. Astringents
   iv. Diagnostic agents
   v. Anticaries and dentifrices
f. Write chemical properties, storage and handling of sodium hydroxide or ammonia strong solution.

Q 2. Answer any *three* of the following:
a. Match the following pairs (A) with (B)

A	B
i. Selenium sulfide	1. Seborrheic dermatitis
ii. Kaolin	2. Antischistosomiasis
iii. Dimethicones	3. Lead limit test
iv. Ringer's solutions	4. Barium sulphate
v. Tartar emetic	5. Silicon polymer
vi. Dithiazone	6. Dusting powder
vii. Diagnostic agent	7. Silver nitrate
viii. Warts	8. Electrolyte replenisher

b. Name the official compounds, write properties and uses of ferrous sulphate.
c. What are electrolyte replenisher? Give an account of sodium chloride and its official preparations or potassium chloride and its official preparations.
d. Explain in brief silicon polymers or expectorants.

Q 3. Answer any *three* of the following:
a. Define emetics. Give properties of inorganic compounds used as emetics.
b. Define antidotes. Name the inorganic antidote for cyanide poisoning. Write its physical, chemical properties and official preparation.

c. Define and give examples of (any *two*):
   i. Respiratory stimulant iii. Official buffers
   ii. Inhalants
d. Give properties and uses of sodium thiosulphate or sulphur dioxide. Mention incompatibilities.

Q 4. Answer any *three* of the following:
a. Name the compounds used in treatment of constipation. Classify cathartics with examples. Explain mechanism of action of saline cathartics.
b. Name the inorganic compounds used as:
   i. Protectives iii. Antimicrobial
   ii. Astringent
   Mention the official preparations and uses in detail.
c. Define and explain abrasive and dentifrices. Give properties and uses of fluoride types of compound.
d. Fill in the blanks:
   i. Milk of magnesia is stabilised by addition of _____.
   ii. _____ paper is turned brown red, when dipped in aqueous solution of _____.
   iii. Very dilute solution of HCl is used in _____.
   iv. Aluminum phosphate is _____.
   v. Chemically talc is _____.
   vi. Sodium citrate is _____ for blood.
   vii. Zinc sulphate is ophthalmic _____.

Q 5. Answer any *three* of the following:
a. Give official procedure of limit test for chloride and sulphate.
b. Give types and sources of impurities in pharmaceuticals.
   Or Explain volumetric methods of analysis used for quantity control of compounds.
c. Give medicinal uses of (any *four*):
   i. Calcium carbonate
   ii. Bismuth subcarbonate
   iii. Titanium dioxide
   iv. Potassium permanganate
   v. Kaolin
   vi. Zinc oxide
d. Give properties and uses of following compounds (any *two*):
   i. Boric acid iii. Copper sulphate
   ii. Ammoniated mercury iv. Iodine

Q 6. Answer any *three* of the following:
a. Name the compounds used to treat (any *eight*):
    i. Urticaria   vi. Dysentery
    ii. Scabies   vii. Pruritis
    iii. Hyperthyroidism   viii. Flatulence
    iv. Asthma   ix. Polycythemia vera
    v. Arthritis
b. Give properties and uses of (any *two*):
    i. Hydrogen peroxide
    ii. Magnesium sulphate
    iii. Sodium metabisulfite
c. Mention the advantages and disadvantages of following compounds as antacids:
    i. Sodium carbonate
    ii. Aluminium hydroxide gel
    iii. Magnesium carbonate
d. Explain the role of sodium, potassium and chloride in the body. What is replacement therapy?

Summer Examination 1998
D Pharm First Year
Pharmaceutical Chemistry I

Q 1. Attempt any *ten* of the following:
a. Explain the following terms (any *two*):
    i. Inhalants   iii. Preservatives
    ii. Adsorbents
b. Define and classify the topical agents.
c. Give the synonyms of the following:
    i. Mercury   iii. Sublimed sulphur
    ii. Borax   iv. Magnesium sulphate
d. Match the following pairs (A) with (B)

A	B
i. Sodium fluoride	1. Desensitizing agent
ii. Strontium chloride	2. Dental cement
iii. Zinc sulphate	3. Anti-infective
iv. Zinc oxychloride	4. Astringent
	5. White vitriol
	6. Mottled enamel

e. Write the incompatibility of the following (any *two*):
   i. Sodium fluoride
   ii. Zinc chloride
   iii. Silver nitrate
f. Write the chemical composition of the following (any *two*):
   i. Sodium meta phosphate
   ii. Alum
   iii. Mild silver protein
g. Write the storage conditions of the following (any *two*):
   i. Iodine IP
   ii. Bleaching powder
   iii. Hydrogen peroxide solution IP
h. Write the physical properties of the following (any *two*):
   i. Potassium permanganate IP
   ii. Dimethicone
   iii. Calamine IP
i. Give the reasons of the following:
   Aqueous solution of iodine is preferred to iodine tincture.
j. State the medicinal uses of following:
   i. Boric acid IP
   ii. Bismuth subcarbonate
k. Define and classify the cathartics with examples.
l. Fill in the blanks:
   i. Sodium nitrite is an antidote for _____ poisoning.
   ii. Boric acid on heating to about 160°C temperature, produces the anhydride of _____.
m. Write the uses of gaseous antioxidants.

Q 2. Solve any *three* of the following:

a. Differentiate the "extracellular fluid" and "intercellular fluid" of body system.
b. Write the characteristics of hyponatremia and hypernatremia.
c. Define mEq/L and calculate the number of mEq of sodium chloride in one liter of 0.90% w/v solution.
d. Explain the role of phosphate in the body fluids.
e. Write the importance of replacement therapy.

Q 3. Attempt any *three* of the following:

a. i. Ferrous salts are preferred to ferric salts for oral supplemental therapy. Explain.
    ii. Dibasic calcium phosphate IP prefers to tribasic calcium phosphate IP in calcium deficiency states.
b. Name the four official compounds of iron. Write the chemical formula and structure of them.

c. Write the properties, uses, storage conditions and incompatibilities of potassium iodide.
d. Calcium gluconate is the drug of choice for severe hypocalcemic tetany. Discuss.

Q 4. Attempt any *three* of the following:
a. Define:
  i. Isotopes
  ii. Radioisotopes
  iii. Half-life
b. State the half-life of any two radioactive elements. Enlist the various devices used in measurement of radioactivity. Draw well labelled diagram of GM counter.
c. Compare the properties of alpha and gamma rays.
d. Write the properties, uses, route of administration and dose of barium sulphate.

Q 5. Attempt any *three* of the following:
a. Name the various sources of impurities. Discuss how the cross-contamination incorporates impurity.
b. Define (any *four*):
  i. Determinate errors
  ii. Outlier
  iii. Significant figures
  iv. Specificity
  v. LOD
c. Write the procedure for the limit test of chloride for potassium permanganate IP.
d. Write the principle involved in the limit test of arsenic.

Q 6. Attempt any *two* of the following:
a. Give the identification test IP for the following ion/radicals:
  i. Acetate
  ii. Bromides
  iii. Nitrates
b. Write the following chemical reactions (any *three*):
  i. Sodium benzoates warmed with a few drops of sulphuric acid.
  ii. Aqueous solution of bicarbonate boiled with magnesium sulphate.
  iii. Iodide solution treated with potassium iodide solution and dilute acetic acid.
  iv. Aqueous solution of phosphate is mixed with ammonical magnesium sulphate solution.
c. Complete the following reactions and write names of products (any *six*):
  i. $NaHCO_3 + HgCl_2 \longrightarrow$

ii. $NaCl + H_2SO_4 + MnO_2 \longrightarrow$
iii. $KI + K_2Cr_2O_7 + H_2SO_4 \longrightarrow$
iv. $Na_2SO_4 + (CH_3 COO)_2Pb \longrightarrow$
v. $Na^+ + KH_2 SbO_4 \longrightarrow$
vi. $AgCl + K_2CrO_4 \longrightarrow$
vii. $Fe^{+++} + 3K_4 Fe(CN)_6 \longrightarrow$

Winter Examination 1998
D Pharm First Year
Pharmaceutical Chemistry I

Q 1. Attempt any *ten* of the following:

a. Explain the following terms (any *two*)
   i. Achlorhydria
   ii. Astringents
   iii. Emetics

b. Give the synonyms of the following:
   i. Magnesium sulphate
   ii. Sodium bicarbonate
   iii. Kaolin IP
   iv. Borax

c. Match the following pair (A) with (B)

A	B
i. Mild silver protein	1. Antidandruff agent
ii. Silver nitrate	2. Treatment of rhinitis tonsillitis
iii. Zinc sulphate	3. Haemostatic and styptic
iv. Selenium sulphide	4. Photographic film
	5. Prophylaxis of ophthalmia neonatorum

d. Name one compounds from each class (any *two*):
   i. Respiratory stimulant
   ii. Desensitising agent
   iii. Antacid

e. Write the chemical incompatibilities of following (any *two*):
   i. Sodium metabisulphite
   ii. Sodium thiosulphate
   iii. Ammoniated mercury

f. Write the chemical formula of the following:
   i. Sodium potassium tartrate
   ii. Magnesium trisilicate IP
   iii. Sodium tetrathionate
   iv. Sodium metabisulphite IP

g. Write physical properties of following (any *two*):
   i. Calamine IP
   ii. Aluminium hydroxide gel.
   iii. Sodium nitrite
h. Give reasons (any *two*):
   i. Aqueous iodine solution is prefered to tincture of iodine.
   ii. Solution of sodium hydroxide should be stored in hard glass bottles using rubber stoppers.
   iii. Magnesium sulphate acts as saline cathartic on oral administration.
   iv. Define and classify the gastrointestinal agents.
i. Fill in the blanks:
   i. Sodium thiosulphate is an antidote for _____.
   ii. Borate buffers are mixtures of boric acid and _____.
j. Define antioxidants and state the ideal properties for antioxidants.
k. Write the uses of nitrogen.

Q 2. Attempt any *three* of the following:

a. Name the "intra- and extracellular electrolytes". Write the disorders of potassium.
b. Write a note on acid-base regulation by electrolytes.
c. Write the formulation of oral rehydration preparation recommended by UNICEF. State its importance.
d. Define mEq/L. Calculate the number of mEq of sodium chloride in one litre of a 0.90% w/v solution.

Q 3. Attempt any *three* of the following:

a.   i. Explain, ferrous salts are preferred to ferric salts for oral supplemental therapy.
     ii. Explain combination of antacids prefers.
b. Name the four official compounds of calcium. Write the chemical formula and structure of them.
c. Write physical properties, uses, chemical incompatibility and storage conditions of ferrous sulphate IP.
d. Write two pharmaceutical uses and two medicinal uses of following:
     i. Iodine IP   ii. Radioactive iodine

Q 4. Attempt any *three* of the following:

a. Define:
     i. Isotopes   iii. Half-life
     ii. Radioisotopes

b. Compare the properties of alpha and gamma rays.
c. Write the principle involved in the limit test of iron IP 85.
d. Explain the role of radiopaque contrast media.

Q 5. Attempt any *three* of the following:
a. Name the various sources of impurities and write a note on "inadequate storage".
b. Define:
  i. Significant figures
  ii. LOD and LOI
  iii. Desensitizing agents
  iv. Dental fluorosis
c. Draw a well-labelled diagram of Gufzeit test apparatus.
d. The "total quality control in drug industry becomes an organized effort". Explain.

Q 6. Attempt any *two* of the following:
a. Give the identification tests IP for the following ions/radicals.
  i. Benzoate
  ii. Chlorides
  iii. Citrates
b. Write the following chemical reactions (any *three*):
  i. Solution of iodide treated with solution of potassium iodide and dilute acetic acid.
  ii. Aqueous solution of bicarbonate boiled with magnesium sulphate.
  iii. Aqueous solution of phosphate is mixed with ammonical magnesium sulphate solution.
  iv. Sodium acetate is heated with equal quantities of oxalic acid.
c. Complete the following reactions and write the names of products (any *six*):
  i. $CH_3COONa + C_2HOH \xrightarrow{H_2SO_4}$
  ii. $NaCl + H_2SO_4 + MnO_2 \longrightarrow$
  iii. $KI + K_2Cr_2O_7 + H_2SO_4 \longrightarrow$
  iv. $Na + KH_2SbO_4 \longrightarrow$
  v. $AgCl + K_2Cr_2O_4 \longrightarrow$
  vi. $H_2C_2O_4 \cdot 2H_2O + KMnO_4 + H_2SO_4 \xrightarrow{Warm}$
  vii. $Ca(OCl)Cl + CH_3COOH \longrightarrow$

Summer Examination 1999
D Pharm First Year
Pharmaceutical Chemistry I

Q 1. Solve any *five* of the following:
  a. Define radioactivity. Explain biological effects of radiations.
  b. Give formulae, properties and uses of (any *one*):
   i. Talc
   ii. Silicone polymers
  c. Explain achlorhydria. Give its symptoms and name drug used in the treatment of achlorhydria.
  d. Give official procedure of limit test for chloride as per IP 85.
  e. Define anticaries and dentifrices. Give at least two examples of each.
  f. Discuss the properties and uses of povidone iodine. Explain in brief, why it is preferred to iodine.

Q 2. Solve any *three* of the following:
  a. Explain the Arrhenius theory for acids and bases, with its limitations.
  b. Name the different methods for measurement of radioactivity. Draw neat sketch and explain working of GM counter.
  c. Explain the principle involved in the limit test for arsenic with reactions.
  d. Mention anions and cations present in the intra- and extracellular fluids and explain physiology of acid-base balance.

Q 3. Answer any *three* of the following:
  a. Explain the principle of limit test for iron with reactions.
  b. Define laxative, classify them with examples. Give properties and uses of magnesium sulphate.
  c. Give properties, uses and storage conditions of (any *two*):
   i. Potassium permanganate
   ii. Hydrogen peroxide
   iii. Silver nitrate
  d. Explain buffers and their role in pharmaceutical preparations. Mention any one official buffer.

Q 4. Solve any *three* of the following:
  a. Explain raw material and in process quality control.
  b. Explain inhalants function and uses of oxygen.

c. Define hyperacidity and antacids. Give characteristic of ideal antacids. Mention the properties and uses of aluminium hydroxide gel.
d. Explain protective and adsorbents. Give properties and uses of kaolin.

Q 5. Solve any *three* of the following:
a. Explain different types of volumetric methods of analysis.
b. Explain radiopaque contrast media. Give properties and uses of barium sulphate.
c. Give properties, uses and official preparations of sodium chloride.
d. Explain antidote. How do they act? Give properties and uses of sodium thiosulphate.

Q 6. Solve any *three* of the following:
a. Define expectorants and emetics. Give properties and uses of ammonium chloride.
b. Give properties, uses of boric acid and sodium fluoride.
c. Define limit test and tolerable limit. Give composition of barium sulphate reagent. Explain why it is called barium sulphate reagent.
d. Explain ORS powder with its importance. Give at least one formula for ORS mixture.

Winter Examination 1999
D Pharm First Year
Pharmaceutical Chemistry I

Q 1. Solve any *five* of the following:
a. Explain radiopharmaceuticals, give any five applications of radiopharmaceuticals.
b. Give formulae, properties and uses of (any *one*):
  i. Alum
  ii. Sodium potassium tartrate
c. Explain systemic acidosis and alkalosis. Why it causes?
d. Give official procedure of limit test for sulphate as per IP 85.
e. Explain antibacterial action of antimicrobials.
f. Give properties, uses of iodine and silicone polymer.

Q 2. Solve any *three* of the following:
a. Explain the antioxidants, their use in pharmaceutical preparations. Give properties and uses of sodium, metabisulfite.

b. Explain combination of antacid preparation. Give types of antacids, their advantages and disadvantages.
c. Define and explain acids and bases according to Lewis concept and Bronsted and Lowry concept.
d. Explain the electrolytes use for replacement therapy. Give properties, uses and official preparation of potassium chloride.

Q 3. Answer any *three* of the following:
a. Define quality control and quality assurance.
b. Define radioactivity. Give properties of alpha, beta and gamma rays.
c. Explain anticaries and dentifrices. Give properties, uses of sodium fluoride and calcium carbonate.
d. Give properties, uses and storage conditions of (any *two*):
   i. Sodium hydroxide
   ii. Chlorinated lime
   iii. Povidone-iodine

Q 4. Solve any *three* of the following:
a. Explain the principle involved with reaction in the limit test for sulphate as per IP 85.
b. Classify laxative with examples. Explain the actions of saline cathartics. Give properties and uses of magnesium sulphate.
c. Explain the precautions to be taken while handling and storage of radiopharmaceuticals.
d. Explain respiratory stimulant and inhalants. Give functions and uses of carbon dioxide.

Q 5. Solve any *three* of the following:
a. Draw well labelled diagram of apparatus used in limit test for arsenic and give in brief IP specification of apparatus.
b. Explain oral rehydration salt mixture with its importance and formula given by WHO.
c. Name different types of gastrointestinal agents with examples and give properties and uses of drug used in the treatment of achlorhydria.
d. Explain the effect of radiations on the living cells in detail.

Q 6. Solve any *three* of the following:
a. Define antioxidants. Explain criteria used while selecting antioxidants, giving properties and uses of sodium thiosulphate.
b. Explain the use of protectives and astringents. Give properties and uses of calamine.
c. Explain type and sources of impurities in the pharmaceuticals.

d. Give properties, uses and storage condition of (any *two*):
   i. Sodium bicarbonate
   ii. Mild silver protein
   iii. Precipitated sulphur

Summer Examination 2000
D Pharm First Year
Pharmaceutical Chemistry I

Q 1. Solve any *five* of the following:
   a. Explain biological effects of radiations on human body.
   b. Explain principle involved in the limit test for arsenic with reactions.
   c. Explain the term achlorhydria and hyperchlorhydria, give properties and uses of drug used in the treatment of achlorhydria.
   d. Explain combination therapy of electrolyte infusion. Give two formulations used as combination of electrolyte infusion.
   e. Give official procedure of limit test for sulphate as per IP 85.
   f. Define inhalants, explain role of carbon dioxide in the biological system, and give properties and uses of carbon dioxide.
   g. Write the synonyms of:
      i. Borax
      ii. Sublimed sulphur
      iii. Magnesium sulphate
      iv. Mercury

Q 2. Solve any *three* of the following:
   a. Explain, why povidone-iodine is preferred to iodine solution, give properties and uses of povidone-iodine.
   b. Explain respiratory stimulants, give properties and uses of ammonium chloride.
   c. Draw neat sketch, well labelled diagram of GM counter and explain its working.
   d. Explain mechanism of action of antimicrobial agents, give properties and uses of hydrogen peroxide.
   e. Calcium gluconate is the drug of choice for severe hypocalcemic tetany. Explain.

Q 3. Solve any *three* of the following:
   a. Define laxatives, classify them with examples. Explain the action of saline cathartics, give properties and uses of magnesium sulphate.
   b. Explain Arrhenius concept of acid-base with its limitations, give properties and uses of boric acid.

c. Define antacids, classify them with examples, give properties and uses of calcium carbonate.
d. Explain radiopharmaceuticals, give at least six applications of radiopharmaceuticals.
e. Explain the principle of limit test for iron with reactions.

Q 4. Attempt any *three* of the following:
a. Explain topical protectives, give formulae, properties and uses of talc and calamine.
b. Define quality control. Explain inprocess quality control.
c. Give properties, storage conditions and uses of (any *two*):
   i. Magnesium trisilicate
   ii. Sodium thiosulphate
   iii. Alum
d. Explain the term anticaries and dentifrices, give properties and uses of sodium chloride and stannous fluoride.
e. Explain inhalants function and uses of oxygen.

Q 5. Solve any *three* of the following:
a. Explain respiratory and metabolic acidosis and alkalosis.
b. Give official procedure of limit tests for iron as per IP 85.
c. Explain GIT protectives and adsorbents. Give properties and uses of bismuth subcarbonate.
d. Give properties, storage conditions and uses of (any *two*):
   i. Chlorinated lime
   ii. Sodium bicarbonate
   iii. Mild silver protein
e. Explain ORS powder with its importance. Give at least one formula for ORS mixture.

Q 6. Solve any *three* of the following:
a. Define buffers, give types of buffers. Mention official acetate or phosphate buffer.
b. Explain the terms expectorants and emetics, give properties and uses of ammonium chloride.
c. Define antioxidants. Explain its importance. Give properties and uses of sodium metabisulphate.
d. Mention sulphur compounds with their uses, give properties and uses of selenium sulphide.
e. Explain antidotes. How do they act? Give properties and uses of sodium nitrite.

Winter Examination 2000
D Pharm First Year
Pharmaceutical Chemistry I

Q 1. Explain any *five* of the following:
  a. Define the following (any *four*):
     i. Astringents
     ii. Dentifrices
     iii. Emetics
     iv. Hypothyroidism
     v. Contrast media
     vi. Significant figure
     vii. Monograph of drug
  b. Give synonym, formula, properties and uses of (any *one*):
     i. Bismuth subcarbonate
     ii. Antimony potassium tartrate
  c. Give the official procedure of limit test for chloride as per IP 96.
  d. Define and classify antimicrobials; with three examples of each class.
  e. Write properties and uses of iodine and yellow mercuric oxide.
  f. Define "systemic acidosis". Write significance of potassium acetate and sodium citrate.
  g. Write storage conditions and uses of silver nitrate and hydrogen peroxide.

Q 2. Solve any *three* of the following:
  a. Classify antioxidants with two examples of each. Write properties and uses of nitrogen.
  b. Write objectives of combinations of antacids preparations. Write storage conditions of magnesium compounds.
  c. What is achlorhydria? Give the properties and role of an agent used in the treatment of achlorhydria.
  d. What are pharmaceutical buffers? Write names of any three with their significant uses.
  e. Explain protectives and adsorbents. Give properties and uses of calamine.

Q 3. Answer any *three* of the following:
  a. Name electrolytes used in acid-base therapy. Give an account of any one such drug.

b. What are anticaries agents and desensitizing agents. Give properties and storage conditions of zinc chloride and strontium fluoride.
c. Write principle involved in limit test of iron as per IP 96.
d. Explain various sources of impurities. Write a note on "test for as per purity".
e. Write properties, uses and official preparations of sodium chloride.

Q 4. Solve any *three* of the following:

a. Draw a well-labelled diagram for the limit test of arsenic as per IP 96.
b. Define "saline cathartics". Give properties, uses and stability of sodium potassium tartrate.
c. Write construction working and application of GM counter.
d. What are radiopaque? Write properties, uses and storage conditions of barium sulphate.
e. Enlist four official compounds of sodium. Write their chemical formulae and structures.

Q 5. Solve any *three* of the following:

a. Explain respiratory stimulants and inhalants. Give functions and uses of carbon dioxide.
b. Write storage and labelling conditions of nitrous oxide and oxygen.
c. Write a note on storage and handling conditions of radiopharmaceuticals.
d. Discuss the causes of dehydration and functions of electrolytes. Write the formula given by WHO.
e. Name different types of gastrointestinal agents, write examples. Give properties, uses of any one drug used in the diarrhoea.

Q 6. Solve any *three* of the following:

a. Define and classify "antidotes" with examples. Write chemical actions and uses of sodium nitrite.
b. How is the acid-base balance of body maintained?
c. Explain role of iron in the human body. Name three official compounds of iron with their formula.
d. What are radiopharmaceuticals? Write the biological effects of radiations.
e. Write the 'IP identification tests' for the following:
  i. Bromides
  ii. Nitrates

Summer Examination 2001
D Pharm First Year
Pharmaceutical Chemistry I

Q 1. Solve any *five* of the following:
a. Explain Lewis acid-base concept. Give the composition of neutralized phthalate buffer and alkaline borate buffer.
b. Define antioxidants. Give ideal properties of antioxidants and mention uses of sodium nitrate.
c. In a human body, where and which cells secrete hydrochloric acid? Give functions of hydrochloric acid.
d. What are astringents? Explain their uses with examples.
e. Define volume strength. If assay result of hydrogen peroxide sample is 27.5% w/v of H_2O_2, calculate its volume strength.
f. Define the terms isotopes and isobars. Mention the isotopes of carbon and phosphorus.
g. Give official procedure of limit test for chloride as per IP 1996.

Q 2. Solve any *three* of the following:
a. Define the terms—pharmacopoeia, monograph and assay. What are the contents of monograph?
b. What factors must be considered in the selection of a pharmaceutical buffer?
c. Mention the applications of buffers in pharmacy.
d. Classify antioxidants with suitable examples.

Q 3. Answer any *three* of the following:
a. Write the functions of thioglycolic acid in the limit test for iron giving chemical reactions.
b. Describe disorders of GI tract along with their treatment with suitable examples of gastrointestinal agents.
c. Give physical properties and uses of sodium bicarbonate and magnesium trisilicate.
d. Define purgatives. Mention their classes giving suitable examples of each class.

Q 4. Attempt any *three* of the following:
a. What are topical agents? Classify with examples. Define the terms disinfectant and astringent.
b. Explain properties, uses and incompatibilities of $KMnO_4$ or chlorinated lime.

c. Describe official iodine preparations with their medicinal uses.

d. Mention allotropic forms of sulphur and describe properties and uses of selenium sulphide.

Q 5. Answer any *three* of the following:

a. What is the cause of dental caries or tooth decay? Explain the role of fluoride in dental hygiene.

b. Define the terms inhalations and inhalants. Describe the role of O_2 and CO_2 in biological system.

c. Prepare a list of some important antidotes along with the type of poisoning treated by them.

d. What do you understand by the terms—respiratory stimulants, expectorants and emetics. Give properties of any two inorganic expectorants.

Q 6. Solve any *three* of the following:

a. Explain the principle behind the limit test for arsenic.

b. What do you understand by metabolic acidosis and alkalosis? Describe the important functions served by potassium or bicarbonate ions in the human body.

c. Describe commercial formulations of oral rehydration salts.

d. Explain the construction and working of GM counter or scintillation counters.

Winter Examination 2001
D Pharm First Year
Pharmaceutical Chemistry I

Q 1. Solve any *five* of the following:

a. Define radioactivity and give any six properties of alpha, beta and gamma rays.

b. Explain principle involved in the limit test for iron with suitable reactions.

c. Explain GIT protectives and adsorbents with their action, give properties and uses of kaolin.

d. Explain ORS mixture, give two ORS formulae recommended by WHO with importance.

e. Give official procedure of limit test for chloride as per IP 85.

f. Explain inhalants and role of oxygen in the biological systems, give properties and uses of oxygen.

g. Give definitions of:
  i. Astringents
  ii. Antacids
  iii. Buffers
  iv. Antioxidants
  v. Diagnostic agents

Q 2. Solve any *three* of the following:
  a. Draw neat sketch labelled diagram of the apparatus used in limit test for arsenic with its specifications.
  b. Mention six different types of antimicrobial agents. Explain mechanism of action of antimicrobials by oxidation, give properties and uses of potassium permanganate.
  c. Define astringents. Explain the important uses of astringents. Give formula, properties and uses of alum.
  d. Mention various allotropic forms of sulphur, give properties and uses of precipitated and sublimed sulphur.
  e. Give physical properties, IP standard, storage conditions and uses of ammonia solution or hydrogen peroxide.

Q 3. Solve any *three* of the following:
  a. Define antioxidants; give criteria applied for the selection of antioxidants; give properties and uses of sodium thiosulphate.
  b. Explain Bronsted-Lowry and Lewis concept for acid and bases.
  c. Give ideal properties of antacids; explain combination preparations of antacids with their importance.
  d. Explain the precaution to be taken while handling and storage of radiopharmaceuticals.
  e. Define and give examples of (any *two*):
    i. Expectorants
    ii. Inhalants
    iii. Respiratory stimulants

Q 4. Solve any *three* of the following:
  a. Give properties, strong condition and uses of (any *two*):
    i. Silicone polymer
    ii. Iodine
    iii. Calcium carbonate
  b. Define impurity; explain sources of impurities incorporated in pharmaceuticals.
  c. Explain extra and intracellular fluids, give properties and uses of sodium chloride.
  d. Explain the term and mention drugs uses as a desensitizing agents and dentifrice; give properties and uses of zinc chloride.
  e. Define radioactivity. Give properties of alpha, beta and gamma rays.

Q 5. Solve any *three* of the following:
a. Define quality assurance; explain quality control of raw materials.
b. Explain physiological acid-base balance with respiratory acidosis and alkalosis.
c. Give properties, storage conditions and uses of (any *two*):
   i. Talc iii. Silver nitrate
   ii. Hydrogen peroxide
d. Define expectorants and emetics, give properties and uses of potassium iodide.
e. What is calamine and povidone iodine? Give their uses.

Q 6. Solve any *three* of the following:
a. Define 'buffer'. Mention its types, explain in brief official buffers.
b. Explain radiopaque contrast media; give properties and uses of barium sulphate.
c. Define 'antidotes'; mention types of antidotes with examples; give properties and uses of sodium nitrate.
d. Explain topical protectives with their importance; give properties and uses of zinc oxide.
e. Give official preparations and their IP standards of sodium chloride and iodine.

Summer Examination 2002
D Pharm First Year
Pharmaceutical Chemistry I

Q 1. Answer any *five* of the following:
a. What is tooth decay? Make a list of certain inorganic compounds used in dental preparations. Explain uses of calcium monohydrogen phosphate.
b. Explain storage, labelling and uses of oxygen or nitrous oxide.
c. Define the term respiratory stimulants and give properties and uses of ammonium carbonate.
d. Mention safe and effective orally administered expectorants. Write the principle behind the assay of NH_4Cl.
e. Which inorganic compound is used as antischistosomal agent? Give its physical properties and uses.
f. What do you understand by antidotes? Suggest antidotes for fluoride, cyanide and phosphorus poisoning.
g. Give any three IP identification tests for sodium or carbonate ions.

Q 2. Answer any *three* of the following:
a. Explain quality control and quality assurance.
b. Give the principle behind the limit test for sulphate with special reference to barium sulphate reagent as per IP 1985.
c. What are buffers? Give their types and explain mechanism of buffer action with suitable examples.
d. Define and classify inorganic antioxidants. Explain how hypophosphorus acid functions as antioxidant.

Q 3. Answer any *three* of the following:
a. What are disturbances in normal gastric motility? Explain properties and uses of one saline purgative.
b. What do you understand by achlorhydria? Explain the role of HCl in the stomach and its medicinal uses.
c. Give physical properties, storage conditions and uses of sodium bicarbonate and magnesium sulphate.
d. What are the uses of protectives and adsorbents in general? Give properties and uses of kaolin.

Q 4. Answer any *three* of the following:
a. Classify topical agents with examples. Give uses of astringents and explain physical properties of alum.
b. Explain antibacterial action of antimicrobials.
c. Mention IP standards for iodine and describe official iodine solutions.
d. Give properties, uses and storage conditions of (any *two*):
   i. Povidone-iodine
   ii. Chlorinated lime
   iii. Mild silver protein

Q 5. Answer any *three* of the following:
a. Prepare a list of major physiological ions along with their daily body requirement. Calculate mEq/lit of 0.9% w/v solution of NaCl.
b. Explain respiratory acidosis and alkalosis. Why it causes?
c. Explain mechanism which regulatis acid-base balance in human body fluids. Give a formula of rehydration salt mixture suggested by WHO.
d. Describe properties and uses of sodium chloride, sodium acetate and ammonium chloride.

Q 6. Answer any *three* of the following:
a. What is the role of iron and its preparations in human body? Write a chemical reaction when ferrous sulphate is strongly heated.

b. Define the terms radioactivity, isotopes and radionuclides. Give properties of β radiations.
c. Classify radioactivity detecting devices and list the radioisotopes giving their important medicinal uses.
d. Explain barium sulphate as radiopaque contrast media.
e. Explain the assay of boric acid.

Winter Examination 2002
D Pharm First Year
Pharmaceutical Chemistry I

Q 1. Solve any *five* of the following:
a. Explain principle involved in the limit test for iron with suitable reaction.
b. Give the identification tests with the chemical reaction for the following ions/radicals. (Give two tests for each)
    i. Bicarbonate   ii. Calcium
c. Explain biological effects of radiation on human body.
d. Give properties, uses of boric acid and iodine.
e. Explain the following terms:
    i. Normality of a solution   iii. Expectorant
    ii. Acids   iv. Astringents
f. What are antidotes? Give antidotes for fluorides, cyanide and phosphorus poisoning.
g. Give two examples of each of the following:
    i. Antacids   iii. Antioxidants
    ii. Cathartics   iv. Antimicrobials

Q 2. Solve any *three* of the following:
a. Explain radiopaque contrast media; give properties and uses of barium sulphate.
b. Explain type and sources of impurities in the pharmaceuticals.
c. Mention sulphur compounds with their uses, give properties and uses of selenium sulphide.
d. Define buffers, give types of buffers. Mention official phosphate buffers.
e. Give properties, uses and storage conditions of any *two* of the following:
    i. Hydrogen peroxide   iii. Bleaching powder
    ii. Sodium bicarbonate

Q 3. Solve any *three* of the following:
a. Explain respiratory stimulants, give properties and uses of ammonium chloride.
b. Explain electrolytes used for replacement therapy. Give properties, uses and official preparation of sodium chloride.
c. Draw and label the arsenic testing apparatus. Give principle and reactions involved in limit test for arsenic.
d. Define and classify inorganic antioxidants. Give mechanism of action of any one antioxidant.
e. Explain why calcium gluconate is the drug of choice for severe hypocalcemic tetany.

Q 4. Solve any *three* of the following:
a. Explain Bronsted-Lowry and Lewis concept for acids and bases.
b. Explain the precaution to be taken while handling and storage of radiopharmaceuticals.
c Define the terms "radioactivity" and radioisotopes". What is the half-life of radioactive compound. Describe the construction and working of Geiger-Muller counter.
d. Define and explain quality control and quality assurance.
e. Explain principle and reactions involved in assay of boric acid.

Q 5. Solve any *three* of the following:
a. Explain topical protectives, give formula, properties and uses of talc and calamine.
b. Explain the term "anticaries" and dentifrices". Give properties and uses of sodium fluoride and stannous fluoride.
c. Give principle and reaction involved in the limit test for sulphate IP.
d. Compare the properties of α, β and γ radiations.
e. Give properties, storage conditions and uses of (any *two*):
   i. Silver nitrate   iii. Calcium carbonate
   ii. Silicone polymer

Q 6. Solve any *three* of the following:
a. Give official preparation and their IP standards of kaolin and magnesium sulphate.
b. Define "emetics". Give the structure, properties and uses of antimony potassium tartrate.
c. Explain physiological acid-base balance with respiratory acidosis and alkalosis.
d. Explain oral rehydration salt mixture with its importance and formula given by WHO.

e. Give formula and uses of any *two* of the following:
   i. Alum
   ii. Sodium potassium tartrate
   iii. Magnesium hydroxide

Summer Examination 2003
D Pharm First Year
Pharmaceutical Chemistry I

Q 1. Answer any *five* of the following:
   a. What is test for purity? Write significance of following tests on pharmaceuticals:
      i. Test for anions and cations
      ii. Ash values
   b. Explain with examples how following factors are contributing as a source of impurities in pharmaceuticals:
      i. Raw materials
      ii. Adulteration due to storage
   c. Explain the basis for fixing limits of impurities. What are their types?
   d. Explain the reactions and use of reagents in the limit test for heavy metal and iron impurity in pharmaceuticals.
   e. Write sequential steps involved in the limit test for chloride impurity in potassium permanganate sample IP 1996. Explain modification.
   f. Define the terms:
      i. Pharmacopoeia   iii. Radioisotopes
      ii. Assay   iv. Quality assurance
   g. Explain the use of metalochrome indicators with reference to assay of magnesium sulphate. What is EDTA? Give its structure.

Q 2. Answer any *three* of the following:
   a. Explain one chemical reaction of the following type with suitable example.
      i. Neutralization   iii. Precipitation
      ii. Redox   iv. Complexation
   b. Mention name of inorganic compound used in following conditions and explain how it is useful. (Any *two*)
      i. Achlorhydria   iii. Cyanide poisoning
      ii. Dehydration
   c. What precautions will you take during storage and handling of potassium permanganate? Write uses of boric acid and kaolin.

d. Name and write composition of official iodine solutions with their synonyms and uses.
e. Name any two polymerization products. Explain their uses.

Q 3. Answer any *three* of the following:
a. Name the active ingredients of following and explain their use and incompatibilities. (Any *two*)
  i. Styptic pencil
  ii. Calamine
  iii. Barium meal
b. What are advantages of sodium lactate over sodium bicarbonate in treatment of metabolic acidosis? Give their official preparations and uses.
c. Explain dehydration of boric acid and explain use of glycerine in its assay.
d. Explain role of buffers in practice of pharmacy. Write suitable examples.
e. Name the inhalant used to treat hypoxaemia. Write properties and storage of the compound.

Q 4. Answer any *three* of the following:
a. Define:
  i. Half-life of radiopharmaceuticals
  ii. Milli and micro curie
Write about handling and storage of radiopharmaceuticals.
b. Write characteristic of hyponatremia and hypernatremia. What is ORS?
c. Name the inorganic compound with its chemical formula used as:
  i. Emetic   iii. Anticaries
  ii. Antiseborrhoeic   iv. Haemostatic
d. Classify antidotes with examples. Write uses of such compounds.
e. Write identification test for:
  i. Acetate   iii. Aluminum iron
  ii. Bromide

Q 5. Answer any *three* of the following:
a. Write chemical formula, uses and incompatibility of:
  i. Sodium lactate
  ii. Sodium metabisulphate
b. Ferrous salts are preferred to ferric salts for oral supplement therapy, explain.
c. Calcium gluconate is the drug of choice for severe hypocalcemic tetany. Explain. Write its properties and formula.

d. Name the inorganic compound used in treatment of:
   i. Achlorhydria   iii. Diarrhoea
   ii. Dental caries   iv. Ear infections
   Write chemical formula of the above compounds.
e. Write physical properties and uses of (any *two*):
   i. Precipitated sulphur
   ii. Chlorinated lime
   iii. Ammoniated mercury

Q 6. Answer any *three* of the following:
   a. What are expectorants? Write examples of compounds with their uses and incompatibility.
   b. Write properties and uses of (any *two*):
      i. Mild silver protein
      ii. Magnesium sulphate
      iii. Calcium hydroxide
   c. Name the inorganic compound used in or as:
      i. Ulcers
      ii. Preservative
      iii. Cyanide poisoning
      iv. Constipation
      Write properties of any *two* such compounds.
   d. Explain (any *two*):
      i. Use of combination of antacids
      ii. Quality control of pharmaceuticals
      iii. Electrolyte therapy
      iv. Use of protectives
   e. Give an account of antioxidants commonly used. What is the basis of their choice?

Winter Examination 2003
D Pharm First Year
Pharmaceutical Chemistry I

Q 1. Answer any *five* of the following:
   a. Give any three IP identification tests for ferrous (Fe^{++}) and chlorides.
   b. Give properties, uses and storage conditions of:
      i. Hypophosphorus acid
      ii. Potassium iodide
   c. Define half-life of radioelement. Explain working of GM counter.
   d. Give the principle behind chloride limit test IP.

e. Explain formulation of ORS (oral rehydration salt).

f. What is metabolic acidosis and metabolic alkalosis?

Q 2. Answer any *three* of the following:

a. Define radiopaque contrast media. Explain properties and uses of barium sulphate.

b. Explain uses and assay of calcium gluconate.

c. Explain hypothyroidism and give uses and incompatibilities of iodine.

d. Define antimicrobials. Explain preparation, properties and uses of povidone-iodine.

Q 3. Answer any *three* of the following:

a. Define respiratory stimulants and emetics with examples.

b. What is cause of dental caries? Explain role of fluoride in dental hygiene.

c. Define astringent and give properties and uses of zinc sulphate.

d. Give different forms of sulphur and describe properties and uses of selenium sulphide.

Q 4. Answer any *three* of the following:

a. Classify antimicrobials with examples and describe properties, uses and storage of mild silver protein.

b. Explain application of buffers in pharmaceutical preparations.

c. Give sources of impurities in pharmaceutical preparation.

d. Define antacids. Give properties, uses and preparation of milk of magnesia.

Q 5. Answer any *three* of the following:

a. Explain acid-base as per Lewis concept with example.

b. Explain mechanism of action of saline cathartics.

c. Define protectives and adsorbents. Discuss properties and uses of calamine.

d. Give assay, properties and uses of hydrogen peroxide.

Q 6. Answer any *three* of the following:

a. Define antioxidant. Give molecular formula, properties and uses of sodium thiosulphate.

b. What are the applications of gastrointestinal protectives and adsorbents?

c. Draw diagram of Gutzeit apparatus.

d. Which are the commercial preparations of iodine used as antiseptics?

e. Explain quality control and quality assurance.

Summer Examination 2004
D Pharm First Year
Pharmaceutical Chemistry I

Q 1. Solve any *five* of the following:
  a. What are limit tests? Give principle behind limit test for heavy metals.
  b. Discuss the causes of dehydration and functions of electrolytes.
  c. Explain the following terms (any *two*):
     i. Achlorhydria   iii. Astringents
     ii. Emetics
  d. Write chemical incompatibilities of the following (any *two*):
     i. Ammoniated mercury   iii. Sodium metabisulphite
     ii. Sodium thiosulphate
  e. Discuss biological effects of radiation. Write applications of radiopharmaceuticals.
  f. Write chemical properties, storage and handling of sodium hydroxide.
  g. Give official procedure for limit test for sulphate IP.

Q 2. Solve any *three* of the following:
  a. Write objectives of combinations of antacid preparations. Write storage conditions of magnesium compounds.
  b. Define: mEq/L. Calculate the number of mEq of sodium chloride in one litre of 0.90% w/v solution.
  c. Name the intra- and extracellular electrolytes. Write the disorders of potassium.
  d. What are pharmaceutical buffers? Write name of any three with their significant uses.
  e. Give chemical formula, properties and uses of any *two* of the following:
     i. Dicalcium phosphate
     ii. Calcium carbonate
     iii. Sodium metabisulphate

Q 3. Solve any *three* of the following:
  a. Write properties, uses and official preparations of ammonium chloride.
  b. Define topical agents. Classify them giving examples.
  c. Give identification test for the following ions/radicals
     i. Potassium   iii. Chlorides
     ii. Acetate

d. Name four official compounds of calcium. Give their chemical formula and uses.
e. Define and give examples of any *two* of the following:
   i. Inhalants
   ii. Antacids
   iii. Respiratory stimulant

Q 4. Solve any *three* of the following:

a. Name the compounds used in constipation. Classify cathartics with examples. Explain mechanism of saline cathartics.
b. Define (any *two*):
   i. Isotopes
   ii. Radioisotopes
   iii. Half-life
c. Explain properties and uses of oxygen.
d. What are radiopaques? Give properties, action and uses of barium sulphate.
e. Give principle and reaction involved in limit test for iron IP?

Q 5. Solve any *three* of the following:

a. How is the acid–base balance of the body maintained? Give brief account of electrolyte combination therapy.
b. Give principle and procedure for limit test of chloride.
c. Explain the role of iron in the human body. Name two official compounds of iron with their formula and physical properties.
d. What are buffers. Explain the mechanism of action of buffers with suitable example.
e. Write principle and reactions involved in the assay of copper sulphate.

Q 6. Solve any *three* of the following:

a. What are the uses of protectives and adsorbents in general? Give properties and uses of kaolin.
b. Calculate mEq/L of calcium and chloride in the 0.033% $CaCl_2 \cdot 2H_2O$ solution.
   (Given: At. wts. of Ca = 40; Cl = 35.5)
c. Explain mechanism of action of antimicrobials.
d. Define:
   i. LOD and LOI
   ii. Significant figure
   iii. Diagnostic agents
   iv. Dental fluorosis
e. Explain the electrolytes used for replacement therapy. Give properties, uses and official preparations of potassium chloride.

Winter Examination 2004
D Pharm First Year
Pharmaceutical Chemistry I

Q 1. Solve any *five* of the following:
  a. Describe the reactions of boric acid with glycerine.
  b. Mention the precautions, storage conditions of sodium hydroxide and strong ammonia solution.
  c. Explain the necessity, mechanism and criteria of selection in regards of antioxidants.
  d. State the properties of magnesium trisilicate and sodium bicarbonate.
  e. Explain the gastrointestinal disorders and mention the pharmaceuticals used therein.
  f. Give the mechanism by which antimicrobial agents act.
  g. State the properties of two zinc compounds used as topical protectives.

Q 2. Solve any *three* of the following:
  a.   i. Explain the terms with examples—Desensitizing agents, anticaries agents.
      ii. Mention the molecular formula—Magnesium sulphate, calcium hydroxide.
  b. Define topical agents, classify them giving examples.
  c. Explain acid-base as per Lowry-Bronsted theory.
  d. Define the following terms (any *four*):
      i. Inhalants
      ii. Antacid
      iii. Radioisotopes
      iv. Half-life
      v. Achlorhydria
  e. Give the storage of oxygen, carbon dioxide, nitrous oxide and hydrogen peroxide.

Q 3. Solve any *three* of the following:
  a. Give the synonyms of ammonium carbonate, calcium carbonate, antimony, potassium tartrate, hydrochloric acid.
  b. State the properties and uses of sodium nitrite and potassium iodide.
  c. Define buffers and mention their uses in pharmacy.
  d. Discuss the limit test for arsenic and the Gutzeit apparatus.
  e. Write objectives of combination antacid therapy. Write storage conditions for aluminium compounds.

Q 4. Solve any *three* of the following:
a. Describe the major intra- and extracellular physiological ions.
b. Give principle and reactions for limit test for iron.
c. Define mEq/L. Calculate the mEq of sodium chloride in one litre of 0.9% w/v solution.
d. Give the labelling, storage and handling precautions in regards of radiopharmaceuticals.

Q 5. Solve any *three* of the following:
a. Elaborate the role of iron and calcium in physiology along with the list of their official compounds.
b. Give the identification tests for chloride, calcium, potassium, sulphate.
c. State the uses of sodium phosphate P_{32} injection, sodium iodide I_{131} solution, cobalt Co_{60}, Povidone-iodine solution.
d. Give chemical formula and properties for (any *two*):
   i. Dicalcium phosphate   iii. Sodium metabisulphite
   ii. Calcium carbonate
e. State the reactions and explain the principle involved in the assay of hydrogen peroxide solution.

Q 6. Solve any *three* of the following:
a. Give the principle, reaction and procedure involved in the limit test for sulphate.
b. Discuss the different sources by which impurities can enter in pharmaceuticals.
c. Describe the term 'quality', how it can be controlled and what is the importance in doing so.
d. Classify the various cathartics with examples. Explain mechanism of action of saline cathartics.
e. Explain formulation of ORS (oral rehydration salt).

Summer Examination 2005
D Pharm First Year
Pharmaceutical Chemistry I

Q 1. Answer any *five* of the following:
a. Define acid and base as per Arrhenius concept. Give two examples of each.
b. Explain principle involved in iron limit test with reaction involved in it.

c. What is the significance of quality control in pharmaceutical industry?
d. Define antiseptic and disinfectants. Explain properties and uses of silver nitrate.
e. Define antacids. Give properties, uses of aluminium hydroxide gel.
f. Explain reactions involved and procedure of chloride limit test as per IP.
g. Give the preparation, properties and uses of sodium fluoride.

Q 2. Answer any *three* of the following:
a. What criteria should be applied while selecting a suitable antioxidant?
b. Define expectorants and write physical properties, uses, assay of ammonium chloride.
c. Describe official preparations of iodine with its medicinal use.
d. Explain principle involved in assay of boric acid and reactions involved in it.

Q 3. Answer any *three* of the following:
a. Define antidote and classify with examples.
b. Define protectives and adsorbents. Discuss action and uses of kaolin and talc.
c. Define cathartics. Classify with examples.
d. Explain properties and uses of sodium metabisulphite and nitrogen.

Q 4. Answer any *three* of the following:
a. What are the topical agents? Classify with examples.
b. What is achlorhydria? Explain its treatment.
c. Explain role of sodium as major extracellular ion.
d. Draw diagram of Gutzeit apparatus.

Q 5. Answer any *three* of the following:
a. Give molecular formulae of alum borax, sodium thiosulphate and calamine.
b. Explain properties and uses of sodium potassium tartrate.
c. Give the principle behind the limit test for sulphate with special reference to barium sulphate reagent as per IP 1985.
d. Explain role of sodium nitrite in cyanide poisoning.

Q 6. Answer any *three* of the following:
a. Describe physical properties and uses of ferrous sulphate.
b. Define astringent; properties and uses of alum.
c. Define radiopaque contrast media. Explain properties and uses of barium sulphate.

d. Define antimicrobial agents. Explain mechanism by which they act.
e. Give properties, uses and storage conditions of (any *two*):
   i. Hydrogen peroxide   iii. Mild silver protein
   ii. Potassium permanganate

Winter Examination 2005
D Pharm First Year
Pharmaceutical Chemistry I

Q 1. Answer any *five* of the following:
  a. Define the terms:
     i. Buffers
     ii. Quality control and assurance
     iii. X-ray contrast media
     iv. Preservatives
  b. Name the indicators used in complexometric titration. Explain its principle. Write assay method for hydrogen peroxide IP.
  c. How will you perform limit test for chloride impurity in coloured substances? Explain with example.
  d. Explain the reactions involved in limit test for lead and iron impurity.
  e. Absolute purity is difficult and costly. Justify your answer and state sources of impurities.
  f. Define test for purity. Name the various tests performed under this head for pharmaceuticals.
  g. Write assay method for boric acid. What is back titration? Explain with suitable example.

Q 2. Answer any *three* of the following:
  a. Give the classification of various gastrointestinal agents. Name inorganic compounds and their uses.
  b. Name the inorganic compounds used in treatment of:
     i. Achlorhydria   iii. Cyanide poisoning
     ii. Anticaries   iv. Hyperacidity
     Write chemical formula of each compound.
  c. Write physical properties and uses of (any *two*):
     i. Selenium sulphide   iii. Mercury
     ii. Borax
  d. Name the drug of choice in severe hypocalcemic tetany. Write its properties and storage.
  e. Classify laxatives and give advantages and disadvantages of magnesium sulfate.

Q 3. Answer any *three* of the following:
a. Write any two:
   i. Uses of astringents (in which conditions)
   ii. Uses of inhalants (in which conditions)
   iii. Monographs of official drugs
b. What are expectorants and emetics? Give properties and uses of antimony potassium tartrate.
c. Write IP standard, storage and uses of ammonia solution and hydrogen peroxide.
d. Give uses and incompatibility produced by following compounds (any *two*)
   i. Potassium permanganate   iii. Sodium nitrite
   ii. Calcium hydroxide
e. What are antioxidants? Explain the pharmaceutical use with examples of compounds.

Q 4. Answer any *three* of the following:
a. Define mEq. Calculate the mEq of NaCl in one litre of 0.90% w/v solution.
b. Write about storage of radiopharmaceuticals and write two examples along with uses.
c. Write uses of:
   i. Talc   iii. Bismuth subcarbonate
   ii. Titanium dioxide   iv. Zinc oxide
d. Name important official preparations of sodium chloride and iodine.
e. What do you know about polymerization? Write suitable examples along with uses.

Q 5. Answer any *three* of the following:
a. Write active ingredients of the following:
   i. Calamine lotion   iii. Barium meal
   ii. Styptic pencil   iv. Normal saline
   Write chemical formula of these compounds with their uses.
b. Explain action of heat on:
   i. Potassium permanganate   ii. Yellow mercuric oxide
   Write their incompatibility and storage.
c. Name intra- and extracellular electrolytes. Write the disorders of potassium.
d. Why is sodium lactate is preferred to sodium bicarbonate? Write names of their official preparations.
e. Write assay method based on neutralization or complexometric reaction and explain with examples.

Q 6. Answer any *three* of the following:
 a. Write two identification test for (any *two*):
  i. Barium iii. Iodides
  ii. Bismuth
 b. What is hypoxaemia and dehydration? Write properties and storage of compounds used in hypoxaemia and dehydration.
 c. Explain barium sulfate as X-ray contrast medium with its properties, storage and incompatibilities.
 d. What are various dental products? Name the compounds used with their chemical formulae. What is tooth decay?
 e. Write uses of:
  i. Nitrogen
  ii. Radioactive iodine
  iii. Magnesium trisilicate
  iv. Zinc oxychloride

Summer Examination 2006
D Pharm First Year
Pharmaceutical Chemistry I

Q 1. Attempt any *five* of the following:
 a. Define the following terms (any *four*):
  i. Inhalants iv. Emetics
  ii. Isotopes v. Antioxidants
  iii. Half-life
 b. Define buffers and give mechanism of buffer action with suitable example.
 c. Discuss Bronsted and Lowry concept on acids and bases with examples.
 d. Define achlorhydria and give reasons why it occurs, name any agent used in this condition along with its properties.
 e. Explain mechanism of action of inorganic antioxidants. Give two properties and uses of sodium thiosulphate.
 f. Give four properties of an ideal antacids? Describe importance of combination preparation of antacid with its uses.
 g. Describe the reactions of boric acid with glycerine.

Q 2. Solve any *three* of the following:
 a. Write storage, labelling and uses of nitrogen gas.
 b. Define laxatives an classify with examples.

c. Prepare a list of important antidotes along with the type of poisoning treated by them.
d. Define volume strength. If assay result of hydrogen peroxide sample is 27.5% w/v of H_2O_2 calculate its volume strength.
e. Write two properties and uses of the following:
    i. Talc   ii. Kaolin

Q 3. Solve any *three* of the following:

a. Give the meaning of the following conditions.
    i. Metabolic alkalosis
    ii. Dental fluorosis
    iii. Dehydration
    iv. Hyperthyroidism
b. Give the principle and reactions involved in limit test for iron impurities.
c. How is acid-base balance of the body maintained?
d. Give the formula of ORS given by WHO and UNICEF and give use of each ingredient.
e. Why is calcium gluconate the drug of choice for severe hypocalcemic tetany. Give its properties and uses.

Q 4. Solve any *three* of the following:

a. Discuss the limit test for arsenic and draw well-labelled diagram of Gutzeit apparatus.
b. Write four important sources of impurities in pharmaceuticals.
c. Give important properties of α, β and γ radiations and compare them.
d. Write two Indian pharmacopoeial identification tests for the following:
    i. Sodium ion   ii. Carbonate ion
e. Give the synonyms for the following:
    i. Rochelle salt   iii. Magaldrate
    ii. Epsom salt   iv. Barium meal

Q 5. Solve any *three* of the following:

a. How do antimicrobial agents act as bacteriostatic and bactericide. Give its mechanism of action.
b. Why is povidone-iodine preferred to iodine. Give its three properties and uses.
c. Give molecular formula, synonym, properties and uses of antimony potassium tartrate.
d. Give different forms of sulphur and give two properties and uses of selenium sulphide.

e. What are precautions to be taken during the storage, handling of the following:
   i. Sodium hydroxide   ii. Radiopharmaceuticals

Q 6. Solve any *three* of the following:
  a. What are desensitising agents? Give two properties and uses of strontium chloride.
  b. Give four important uses of radiopharmaceuticals.
  c. Write four official preparations of the following:
     i. Iron   ii. Calcium
  d. Write incompatibilities of the following:
     i. Calcium gluconate
     ii. Iron salts
     iii. Hypophosphorus acid
     iv. Potassium iodide
  e. How do sodium nitrite and sodium thiosulphate act as an antidote in cyanide poisoning?

Winter Examination 2006
D Pharm First Year
Pharmaceutical Chemistry I

Q 1. Solve any *five* of the following:
  a. Define Arrhenius acids and bases with examples and discuss the limitations of the theory.
  b. Define any *four* of the following:
     i. Expectorants and emetics
     ii. Antidotes
     iii. Quality assurance
     iv. Milli and micro curie
     v. Dental fluorosis
  c. Discuss the principle and reactions involved in limit test for iron IP.
  d. Discuss the properties, uses, storage condition and handling of potassium permanganate.
  e. Explain "calcium gluconate is the drug of choice for severe hypocalcemic tetany". Mention its properties and formula.
  f. Write chemical incompatibilities for (any *two*):
     i. Hypophosphorus acid   iii. Iodine
     ii. Ferrous sulphate   iv. Potassium iodide
  g. Define topical agents. Classify them with examples.

Q 2. Solve any *three* of the following:
a. Define buffers. Explain the importance of pharmaceutical buffers.
b. Distinguish between the properties exhibited by alpha (α), beta (β) and gamma (γ) radiations.
c. Discuss the effect of heat on boric acid along with its uses in pharmacy.
d. Give synonyms and molecular formula for:
   i. Chlorinated lime
   ii. Magnesium sulphate
   iii. Aluminium potassium sulphate
   iv. Calcium hydroxide
e. Mention the reactions involved in arsenic limit test IP. Draw a labelled diagram of Gutzeit apparatus.

Q 3. Answer any *three* of the following:
a. Discuss the biological role of iron in the body. Enlist the various official compounds and preparations of iron.
b. Give the mechanism of action and criteria for selection of inorganic antioxidants.
c. Give function of electrolytes. Calculate the mEq of sodium chloride in one litre of 0.9% w/v solution.
d. Give identification tests with reactions for the following ions/ radicals (any *two*).
   i. Chlorides   iii. Potassium
   ii. Sulphates
e. Discuss the objectives of "combination antacid therapy". Discuss the mechanism of action of calcium containing antacids.

Q 4. Answer any *three* of the following:
a. Enlist the various sources of impurities present in pharmaceuticals. How does inadequate storage affect purity of pharmaceuticals?
b. Discuss the role of sodium as a major extracellular ion along with the disorders.
c. Discuss the various precautions for storage and handling of radiopharmaceuticals.
d. Name the inorganic compound used for and write properties of any two such compounds.
   i. Ulcers   iii. Disinfectant
   ii. Topical protective   iv. Emetics
e. Discuss the various gastrointestinal disorders and mention the pharmaceuticals used therein.

Q 5. Answer any *three* of the following:
a. Write properties and uses of (any *two*):
   i. Hydrogen peroxide   iii. Sodium thiosulphate
   ii. Ferrous sulphate
b. Define 'radioactivity'. Discuss radiopaque contrast media with the help of examples.
c. Discuss the biological role of oxygen, Give properties and uses of oxygen.
d. Define astringents and discuss the uses of the astringents.
e. Explain the principle involved in assay of boric acid along with the reactions.

Q 6. Answer any *three* of the following:
a. Discuss the importance of quality control in pharmacy.
b. Classify the various antidotes with examples from each. Write properties and uses of sodium nitrite.
c. Explain ORS powders recommended by WHO with examples.
d. Give the principle, reaction and procedure involved in the limit test for sulphate.
e. Explain the following terms with any two examples (any *two*):
   i. Desensitizing agents   iii. Anticaries agents
   ii. Respiratory stimulants   iv. Reducing agents

Summer Examination 2007
D Pharm First Year
Pharmaceutical Chemistry I

Q 1. Solve any *five* of the following:
a. Define the following terms (any *two*):
   i. Haematinics   iv. Expectorants
   ii. Inhalants   v. Desensitizing agents
   iii. Emetics
b. Write the incompatibilities of the following:
   i. Sodium nitrite   iii. Potassium iodide
   ii. Ferrous sulphate iv. Ammonium chloride
c. What are antidotes? Classify with examples and give use of sodium nitrite.
d. Give synonym, formula, properties, uses, storage and handling of sodium hydroxide.
e. Give the principle of arsenic limit test.

    f. Define mEq. Calculate the mEq of NaCl in one litre of 1.6% w/v of solution.

    g. How are impurities incorporated in pharmaceutical substances?

Q 2. Solve any *three* of the following:

    a. Describe the use of following reagents in identification tests:
        i. Silver nitrate   ii. Barium chloride

    b. Describe the properties and applications of buffers in pharmacy.

    c. What are antacids? Give important properties of an ideal antacid.

    d. What is dental caries? Explain the role of fluorides in it.

    e. Give the synonyms for the following:
        i. Calcium carbonate
        ii. Zinc sulphate
        iii. Boric acid
        iv. Antimony potassium tartrate

Q 3. Solve any *three* of the following:

    a. Give official procedure of sulphate limit test IP 96 and explain BSR.

    b. Define cathartics and classify with examples.

    c. Define official preparations of iodine with their medicinal uses.

    d. What factors must be considered in the selection of an antioxidant and name two antioxidants.

    e. Explain the terms metabolic acidosis and alkalosis. How are these corrected?

Q 4. Solve any *three* of the following:

    a. What are astringents? Explain their uses/actions.

    b. Discuss Bronsted and Lowry concept on acids and bases with examples. And list limitations of Arrhenious theory.

    c. Write properties and uses of the following:
        i. Kaolin
        ii. Bismuth subcarbonate

    d. Write the role of thioglycolic acid in the iron limit test giving chemical reactions.

Q 5. Solve any *three* of the following:

    a. Explain the following:
        i. Significant figures   ii. Quality control

    b. Define and classify topical agents with examples. Give the uses of calamine.

    c. What are radiopaque compounds? Give properties and uses of any one such compound.

d. Give the molecular formula and uses of:
   i. Sodium metabisulphite
   ii. Nitrous oxide
   iii. Sodium metaphosphate
   iv. Hypophosphorus acid
e. Describe the role of iodine in biological system. Make a list of official compounds of calcium.

Q 6. Solve any *three* of the following:
a. Discuss the biological effects of radiations.
b. Explain the construction and working of GM counter.
c. Write properties, uses, official preparations of sodium chloride.
d. Give different alltropic forms of sulphur and give properties and uses of sublimed sulphur.
e. Name the inorganic compound used for:
   i. Dandruff
   ii. Achlorhydria
   iii. Hypoxia
   iv. Sun burns
   v. Warts
   vi. Peptic ulcer
   vii. Eczema
   viii. Eye infections

Winter Examination 2007
D Pharm First Year
Pharmaceutical Chemistry I

Q 1. Solve any *five* of the following:
a. Define the following terms (any *four*):
   i. Buffer capacity
   ii. Quality control
   iii. Emollients
   iv. Radioisotopes
   v. Keratolytics
b. Define acid and base as Arrhenius and list the limitations of Arrhenius theroy.
c. What are antioxidants? Give mechanism of action of antioxidants with examples.
d. Mention the drawbacks of antacid therapy.
e. Write uses and actions of astringents.
f. What is the significance of quality control in pharmaceutical industry?
g. Write the reactions taking place in arsenic limit test.

Q 2. Solve any *three* of the following:

a. Name one inorganic compound for each class:
   i. Respiratory stimulant   iii. Expectorant
   ii. Desensitising agent   iv. Scabies
b. Name the inorganic compound used in following:
   i. Ulcers   iii. Eye infection
   ii. Filter aids   iv. Dandruffs
c. Give synonyms of the following:
   i. Borax   iii. Sodium hydroxide
   ii. Bleaching powder   iv. Precipitated sulphur
d. Enlist four official compounds of sodium with uses.
e. Write the medicinal uses of:
   i. Magnesium trisilicate   iii. Sodium fluoride
   ii. Zinc chloride   iv. Ca_{44} and Ca_{45}

Q 3. Solve any *three* of the following:

a. Write the chemical formulae of:
   i. Sodium metabisulphite
   ii. Sodium tetrathionate
   iii. Sodium potassium tartrate
   iv. Epsom salt
b. How will you carry out limit test for chloride in case of $KMnO_4$ sample according to IP 96 and give the principle involved in limit test for chloride.
c. Give storage conditions of the following:
   i. $AgNO_3$ iii. $FeSO_4$
   ii. H_2O_2 iv. CO_2 gas
d. Give method of preparation of "milk of magnesia."
e. Define topical agents. Write mechanism of action of antimicrobials and give example.

Q 4. Solve any *three* of the following:

a. Write the principle and reactions involved in limit test for sulphates according to IP 1985 and explain BSR.
b. How much of $CaCl_2$ as dihydrate will be needed to prepare 1 litre of solution containing 10 mEq Ca^{++}/litre.

$$Ca^{++} = 40.08, Cl^- = 35.45$$

c. What is PPM? How will you prepare 20 PPM KCl solution?
d. What are different types of laxatives? Discuss the mechanism of action of "saline cathartics."
e. Give the important function of sodium and potassium ion in the body.

Q 5. Solve any *three* of the following:
  a. Define:
      i. Abrasive   iii. Anticaries agent
      ii. Desensitising agent   iv. Dental fluorosis
  b. Mention different conditions under which oxygen is required to the body. Give medicinal uses of CO_2.
  c. Classify antidotes. Write mechanism of action of cyanide poisoning.
  d. What are expectorants and emetics? Write the mechanism of action of expectorants.
  e. What are metabolic acidosis and alkalosis? How are they corrected (treated)?

Q 6. Solve any *three* of the following:
  a. What are the precautions to be taken in handling and storage of radiopharmaceuticals?
  b. What will happen when boric acid is heated at different temperatures? And write its chemical reactions with glycerine.
  c. Enlist four methods for measurement of radioactivity. Explain photographic plate method or GM counter.
  d. Give major advantages as an antimicrobial agent of povidone iodine over elemental iodine solutions.
  e.   i. Write concentration of 1 ml of std solution of iron used in limit test IP 1985.
      ii. What is the usual limit for heavy metals according to IP.

Summer Examination 2008
D Pharm First Year
Pharmaceutical Chemistry I

Q 1. Solve any *five* of the following:
  a. Define the following terms (any *four*):
      i. Expectorants   iv. Desensitizing agents
      ii. Astringents   v. Radiopaque
      iii. Impurities
  b. Explain mechanism of action of antimicrobial agents by oxidation, halogenation and protein precipitation
  c. Explain achlorhydria, give properties, uses of agent used to treat achlorhydria.
  d. Define acid-base as per Arrhenius concept. Give two examples of each.

e. Explain principle involved in the limit test for iron with reactions involved in it.

f. Define antacids, give types of antacid drugs with examples, properties and uses of aluminium hydroxide gel.

g. Define mili equivalent per litre, calculate mEq of sodium chloride in one litre of 0.9% (At. wt. of sodium 23 and chloride −35.5).

Q 2. Solve any *three* of the following:

a. Explain the importance of ORS mixture, give two formulas recommended by WHO and UNICEF.

b. Draw neat sketch labelled diagram and explain working of GM counter.

c. Define radioactivity and explain six properties of α, β, and γ radiation.

d. Define antioxidants, give criteria for selection of antioxidant.

e. Define inhalants. State the storage conditions for oxygen, carbon dioxide and nitrous oxide.

Q 3. Solve any *three* of the following:

a. Explain rational behind combination, preparations of antacids with examples.

b. Give properties and uses of (any *two*):
   i. Hydrogen peroxide
   ii. Sodium bicarbonate
   iii. Calcium carbonate

c. Define astringents, mention important uses of astringents and properties and uses of alum.

d. Explain intra- and extracellular fluids with diagram and name four major anions and cations.

e. Explain how physiological acid–base balance is maintained of body (mechanisms).

Q 4. Solve any *three* of the following:

a. Define antiseptics and disinfectants. Give properties and uses of povidone-iodine.

b. Explain biological effects of radiations. Explain principle involved in the limit test for arsenic reactions.

c. Explain anticaries and dentifrices, give properties and use of sodium fluoride.

d. Give the molecular formula and synonyms for the following:
   i. Bleaching powder   iii. Laughing gas
   ii. Epsom salt   iv. Baking soda

Q 5. Solve any *three* of the following:
a. Explain the terms cathartics and laxative. Classify laxatives with examples, give uses of magnesium sulphate.
b. Explain radiopharmaceuticals and radioisotopes, give at least two uses/applications of radioisotopes.
c. Explain allotropic forms of sulphur. Give properties and uses of selenium sulphide.
d. Give properties, uses and functions of carbon dioxide and oxygen.
e. Explain the role of iron or Iodine in the body.

Q 6. Solve any *three* of the following:
a. Define antidotes. Explain types of antidotes with examples, give properties and uses of sodium nitrite.
b. Draw well labelled diagram and give specification of apparatus used in limit test for arsenic.
c. Explain four sources of impurities in pharmaceuticals.
d. Define respiratory stimulants and expectorants, give properties and uses of ammonium carbonate.
e. Write two identification tests for the following:
  i. Chloride iron
  ii. Calcium iron

Winter Examination 2008
D Pharm First Year
Pharmaceutical Chemistry I

Q 1. Solve any *five* of the following:
a. Give the molecular formula and synonyms of following compounds:
  i. Sodium thiosulphate
  ii. Borax
  iii. Chlorinated lime
  iv. Sodium bicarbonate
b. Define following terms with examples:
  i. Achlorhydria
  ii. Expectorant
  iii. Antacid
  iv. Laxative
c. Describe the principle behind the limit test for sulphate and add a note on barium sulphate reagent.
d. List four important properties of an ideal antioxidant and give the properties of hypophosphorus acid and strong ammonia solution.
e. Define acid and base as per Lewis theory. Give four important properties of buffer solution.
f. Draw the neat labelled diagram of Gutzeit apparatus with all specifications as per IP.

g. Give reactions of boric acid when,
   i. heated at 100°C, 160°C and above
   ii. with glycerine

Q 2. Solve any *three* of the following:

a. Classify antacids and explain the rational behind combination of antacid preparations with example and reasons.
b. Mention about the mechanism by which the following drugs act as purgatives:
   i. Senna
   ii. Methyl cellulose
   iii. Liquid paraffin
   iv. Magnesium sulphate
c. Define antimicrobial agents and explain three mechanisms of antimicrobial action.
d. Write the properties and uses of the following:
   i. Hydrogen peroxide
   ii. Potassium permanganate
e. Explain the role of sulphur compounds in skin diseases. Give the molecular formula and uses of selenium sulphide.

Q 3. Solve any *three* of the following:

a. Explain the role of fluorides in dental caries. Define desensitising agents with two examples.
b. Define and classify antidote with examples. Name two antidotes used in cyanide poisoning.
c. Mention the uses and storage conditions for:
   i. Oxygen   ii. Carbon dioxide
d. Describe the principle involved in limit test for iron with reactions and reasons.
e. List four sources and four types of impurities in pharmaceutical substances.

Q 4. Solve any *three* of the following:

a. Define topical agents and classify with examples. Give the uses of calamine.
b. Write the properties and uses of:
   i. Ammonium chloride   ii. Potassium iodide
c. Define mEq/L. Calculate the number of mEq of sodium chloride in one litre of 0.9% w/v solution.
d. Explain how physiological acid-base balance is maintained in body?
e. Define metabolic acidosis and alkalosis. Give the reasons for their occurrence. Name the electrolytes used for treatment.

Q 5. Solve any *three* of the following:
   a. What are the inherent drawbacks and incompatibilities of iron compounds? Name two with advantages.
   b. Give one use (category) and synonyms of the following:
      i. Barium sulphate   iii. Ferrous sulphate
      ii. Zinc sulphate   iv. Sodium chloride
   c. Describe the role of iodine in the body.
   d. Give the meaning of following conditions (any *four*)
      i. Tetany   iv. Osteomalacia
      ii. Milk alkali syndrome   v. Hyperkalemia
      iii. Anaemia
   e. Name four devices used for measurement of radiation. Explain GM counter.

Q 6. Solve any *three* of the following:
   a. Define with examples:
      i. Radioisotopes   iii. Radiopharmaceuticals
      ii. Curie   iv. Radiopaque contrast media
   b. Give two identification tests for the following ions:
      i. Chloride   ii. Calcium
   c. Mention four important functions for each:
      i. Sodium ion
      ii. Calcium ion in the body
   d. Write the molecular formula and category of the following (any *two*):
      i. Ferrous sulphate   iii. Sodium fluoride
      ii. Calcium gluconate
   e. Describe the principle involved in limit test for heavy metals, give reasons for acetic acid and explain what is ppm.

Summer Examination 2009
D Pharm First Year
Pharmaceutical Chemistry I

Q 1. Solve any *five* of the following:
   a. Define and classify antioxidants with examples. Give the properties and uses of sodium thiosulphate.
   b. Write cautions to be taken during handling of strong ammonia preparation. Write storage conditions and uses of boric acid.
   c. Write synonym, properties, uses and storage conditions of calcium hydroxide.

d. Define buffer solutions with properties and in brief, comment on role of buffers in pharmacy field.
e. Explain properties, uses, storage conditions and molecular formula of hydrogen peroxide.
f. What are saline cathartics and laxatives? Explain their types of action with examples.
g. Name the inorganic pharmaceuticals used in treatment of mild diarrhoea. Write properties of any two such compounds.

Q 2. Solve any *three* of the following:
a. Write properties and uses of:
  i. Aluminium hydroxide gel   ii. Magnesium oxide
b. Define and write examples of compounds
  i. Achlorhydria   iii. Expectorants
  ii. Antacid   iv. Haematinics
c. Write six ideal characteristics that antacid preparations should satisfy. Write about combination of antacids.
d. Write chemical formula, uses and general information about silicon polymers.
e. Write different mechanisms of antidote action. Write about cyanide poisoning and its treatment.

Q 3. Solve any *three* of the following:
a. Write chemical formula and uses of:
  i. Ammoniated mercury   iii. Stannous fluoride
  ii. Potassium acetate   iv. Alum
b. Explain the terms with examples of compounds:
  i. Antacaries agent   iii. Astringents
  ii. Desensitizing agent iv. Emetics
c. Write uses, chemical and physical properties of the following compounds:
  i. Potassium permanganate   ii. Zinc sulfate
d. Write principle and chemical reactions involved in the limit test for iron impurity in pharmaceuticals.
e. Explain uses, advantages of calcium gluconate and its preparations.

Q 4. Solve any *three* of the following:
a. What are inhalants? Mention uses properties and storage condition of any one compound.
b. Enlist official preparations of sodium chloride with their uses. Write importance of sodium ion in the body fluids.
c. What are principle disorder of acid base imbalance? Mention compounds use in the treatment of metabolic acidosis.

d. Write uses of the following:
   i. Sodium iodide I_{131} solution
   ii. Sodium phosphate P_{32} injections
e. Write biological effects of radiations and uses of barium sulfate.

Q 5. Solve any *three* of the following:
a. Name the official preparations of iron with uses and drawbacks of each.
b. Explain principle involved in limit test of arsenic.
c. Write in detail about four official preparations of iodine.
d. What are the sources of impurities in pharmaceutical substances? Explain four.
e. How is limit test for chloride impurity performed? Comment on modification of test if given sample is $KMnO_4$.

Q 6. Solve any *three* of the following:
a. Mention properties and uses of iodine and ferrous sulfate.
b. Comment on the role of iron in body.
c. Write about measurement of radioactivity.
d. Give advantages of sodium lactate over sodium bicarbonate IV fluids. Give formula of ORS.
e. Define the terms:
   i. Contrast media   iii. Incompatibility
   ii. Limit test   iv. Respiratory stimulants

Summer Examination 2010
D Pharm First Year
Pharmaceutical Chemistry I

Q 1. Solve any *five* of the following:
a. Define buffers and discuss mechanism of buffer action with suitable examples. Mention two pharmaceutical buffers.
b. Discuss Bronsted and Lowry concept of acids and bases with examples. Write uses of boric acid and calcium hydroxide.
c. Define the following terms (any *four*):
i. Slaking   ii. Astringents
iii. Expectorants   iv. Half-life
v. Isotopes
d. Discuss the importance of quality control in pharmaceutical industry.
e. Discuss the mechanism of action of antioxidants and the factors to be considered for selection of a suitable antioxidant.

f. Explain the principle involved in the assay of boric acid with reactions.
g. Mention molecular formula for (any *four*):
   i. Bleaching powder   ii. Calomel
   iii. Borax   iv. Slaked lime
   v. Green vitriol

Q 2. Solve any *three* of the following:
a. Discuss the properties required of an ideal antacid. Enlist the various aluminium containing antacids used.
b. Explain the mechanism of action of "Saline cathartics". Mention synonym, properties and molecular formula for magnesium sulphate.
c. Write two properties and uses of:
   i. Talc   ii. Kaolin
d. Write storage, labelling and uses of oxygen gas.
e. What are the storage conditions and uses for:
   i. Sodium hydroxide
   ii. Hydrogen peroxide

Q 3. Solve any *three* of the following:
a. Classify topical agents with examples. Explain the terms "Antiseptics and Disinfections"
b. Why povidone-iodine is preferred to iodine? Mention properties and uses of povidone-iodine.
c. Explain the terms with examples:
   i. Desensitizing agents
   ii. Anticaries agents
   iii. Radio-opaque contrast media
   iv. Emetics
d. Define "Volume strength" of hydrogen peroxide. Calculate the volume strength of 27.5% w/v solution of hydrogen peroxide.
e. Discuss the various uses of astringents. Mention molecular formula and uses of zinc sulphate and alum.

Q 4. Solve any *three* of the following:
a. Discuss the various fluid compartments of human body. Enlist the functions of sodium ions in the body.
b. Discuss "Electrolyte combination therapy". Explain the term 'ORS' with a suitable example.
c. Give properties and uses of:
   i. Ferrous gluconate
   ii. Calcium gluconate

d. Mention properties, uses, storage and incompatibilities of iodine.
e. Give two identification test for:
   i. Chloride ion
   ii. Lead ion

Q 5. Solve any *three* of the following:
a. Discuss the effects of impurities present in pharmaceuticals.
b. Explain the importance of use of the following reagents:
   i. Thioglycollic acid in iron limit test.
   ii. Barium chloride in sulphate limit test.
   iii. Potassium cyanide in lead limit test.
   iv. Silver nitrate in chloride limit test.
c. Explain how cyanide poisoning can be treated? Mention uses of activated characoal and disodium calcium EDTA.
d. Write the various reactions involved in Arsenic limit test and iron limit test.
e. Give synonyms of:
   i. Antimony potassium tartarate
   ii. Hydrochloric acid
   iii. Copper sulfur
   iv. Sublimed sulfur.

Q 6. Solve any *three* of the following:
a. Discuss labelling, storage and handling precautions in regards of radiopharmaceuticals.
b. Give uses of:
   i. Ca^{44} and Ca^{45}
   ii. N^{13} and N^{15}
   iii. Fe^{55} and Fe^{59}
   iv. Co^{57}
c. Enlist the various units used to measure radioactivity.
d. Calculate the number of mEq. of sodium chloride in one litre of a 0.45%. w/v solution.
e. Explain principle and working of Geiger—Muller counter.

Winter Examination 2010
D Pharm First Year
Pharmaceutical Chemistry I

Q 1. Solve any *five* of the following:
a. Define and classify topical agents with examples.
b. State the uses and properties of Calamine and Silicones.
c. Discuss the storage conditions of Potassium permanganate and hydrogen peroxide.

140 Pharmaceutical Chemistry I

d. Explain the various preparations of iodine.
e. Comment on the reactions:
  i. Ammoniated mercury on heating with Sod-hydroxide.
  ii. Chlorinated lime treated with acetic acid.
f. Give the properties and uses of any one allotropic form of sulphur.
g. Define 'astringents' and mention their uses.

Q 2. Solve any *three* of the following:
  a. Define 'buffer' and explain its role in pharmacy.
  b. Mention the properties of hydrochloric acid and ammonium hydroxide.
  c. Explain the dehydration of boric acid on heating and precautions to be taken in handling of sodium hydroxide.
  d. Explain the terms 'anti-caries' and 'desensitizing agents' with examples.
  e. State the properties of calcium carbonate and sodium phosphate.

Q 3. Solve any *three* of the following:
  a. Give the mechanism by which antioxidants act and mention the properties of sulphur dioxide.
  b. Comment on 'achlorhydria' and hyperhydrochloric dyspepsia'.
  c. Mention the different types of cathartics and properties of Sodium potassium tartrate.
  d. Explain the merits of combining antacids.
  e. Define 'internal protectives' and mention the properties of Bismuth sub-carbonate.

Q 4. Solve any *three* of the following:
  a. Define 'respiratory stimulant' and state the properties of ammonium carbonate.
  b. Mention the uses of carbon dioxide and nitrous oxide.
  c. Define 'expectorants' and give the properties of potassium iodide.
  d. State the storage conditions, precautions and uses of oxygen.
  e. Define 'antidote' and state the properties and uses of sodium nitrite.

Q 5. Solve any *three* of the following:
  a. Explain two principle anions and cations present in extra-and intracellular fluid.
  b. Comment on physiological acid–base balance.
  c. What is oral rehydration? Give details of pharmaceutical formulations available.
  d. Draw a neat labelled diagram of 'Geiger-Muller Counter' and mention the biological effects of radiation.
  e. Define "Radio-opaque contrast media" and give properties of barium sulphate.

Q 6. Solve any *three* of the following:
  a. Define 'impurity' and explain its effect on pharmaceutical preparations.
  b. Give the principle and reaction involved in limit test for iron and chloride.
  c. Draw a neat labelled diagram of Gutzeit test apparatus and reactions involved in limit test for arsenic.
  d. Mention identification test for—Acetate, ammonium, barium and carbonate ions.
  e. Describe the role of calcium or iron in human physiology with special mention of their official preparations.

Summer Examination 2011
D Pharm First Year
Pharmaceutical Chemistry I

Q 1. Answer any *five* of the following:
  a. Explain Arrhenius concept of acid-base with examples. Give properties and uses of strong ammonium hydroxide.
  b. Define the term "Anticaries agent". Give the properties and medicinal uses of sodium fluoride.
  c. What are antidotes? Classify antidotes with examples.
  d. Define—"emetics". Give the chemical formula, properties and category of antimony potassium tartrate.
  e. What are radio-opaque contrast media? Give the properties of barium sulphate.
  f. Give the properties of talc and silicone polymers.
  g. Write the synonyms of:
     i. Precipitated sulphur   ii. Barium meal
     iii. Yellow mercuric oxide   iv. Calcium hydroxide.

Q 2. Answer any *three* of the following:
  a. What is quality control? Discuss importance of quality control in pharmaceutical industry.
  b. Define inhalants. Give the properties and uses of oxygen.
  c. Give the properties, uses of calcium gluconate.
  d. Give the properties and uses of selenium sulphide.

Q 3. Answer any *three* of the following:
  a. Enlist the various source of impurities. Explain the source—"Raw materials".
  b. Define—"Expectorants". Give the properties and uses of ammonium chloride.

c. Give the identification tests with chemical reactions for the following ions/radicals (any *two*):
   1. Acetates
   2. Bicarbonates
   3. Chlorides
d. Write the principle and procedure involved in the limit test for chloride as per I.P.—1996.

Q 4. Answer any *three* of the following:
   a. What are antioxidants? Classify its mechanism with example.
   b. How physiological acid–base balance of the body is maintained? Explain respiratory mechanism.
   c. What is achlorhydria? Give the properties and uses of the agent used in the treatment of achlorhydria.
   d. Write a brief account of ammonium carbonate as a respiratory stimulant.

Q 5. Answer any *three* of the following:
   a. What are antacids? Give the properties and category of aluminium hydroxide gel.
   b. Write the properties of ideal antacid. Classify antacid with example.
   c. Draw neat sketch, well labelled diagram of G.M. counter and explain its working.
   d. Classify saline cathartic with example.

Q 6. Answer any *three* of the following:
   a. Give the properties and storage condition of hydrogen Peroxide and potassium permanganate.
   b. Describe physical properties, method of preparation and category of ferrous sulphate.
   c. What are astringent? Give properties and uses of alum.
   d. Write biological effect of radiation.

Winter Examination 2011
D Pharm First Year
Pharmaceutical Chemistry I

Q 1. Solve any *five*:
   a. Discuss Bronsted and Lowry concept of acids and bases with examples. Write uses of boric acid and calcium hydroxide.
   b. Define "Astringents" and mention their pharmaceutical uses.
   c. Explain the principle and reactions involved in the assay of boric acid.

d. Discuss the properties, uses, storage conditions and handling of chlorinated lime.
e. Explain the significance of quality control in pharmaceutical industry.
f. Explain principle involved in the limit test for Heavy metal with reactions.
g. Define expectorants. Write mechanism of expectorants.

Q 2. Solve any *three*:
 a. Write two properties and uses of the following:
  i. Talc ii. Kaolin
 b. Explain the importance of ORS mixture and give formulas recommended by WHO and UNICEF.
 c. Name one inorganic compound for each class:
  i. Respiratory stimulant ii. Scabies
  iii. Desersitizing agent iv. Dental caries
 d. Classify antacids with examples. Write properties of ideal antacids.
 e. Explain the objectives of 'combination antacid therapy'. Write properties of aluminium hydroxide and sodium bicarbonate.

Q 3. Solve any *three*:
 a. Give the synonyms of:
  i. Antimony potassium tartarate
  ii. Sodium potassium tartarate
  iii. Calcium carbonate
  iv. Hydrochloric acid
 b. Define 'Topical agents'. Classify them with examples.
 c. Discuss the mechanism of action of antioxidants. Mention molecular formula of sodium metabisulphite and sodium nitrite.
 d. Explain mechanism of action of saline cathartics. Mention synonym and molecular formula of magnesium sulphate.
 e. Mention different allotropic forms of sulphur. Write properties and uses of selenium sulphide.

Q 4. Solve any *three*:
 a. Define buffers. Explain the importance of buffers in pharmacy.
 b. Define antidotes. Classify them with examples.
 c. Discuss properties, uses, storage and labelling of nitrous oxide.
 d. Define the following:
  i. Radioisotopes ii. Half-life
  iii. Curie iv. Inhalants
 e. Explain the labelling, storage and handling precautions in regards of radioisotopes.

Q 5. Solve any three:
a. State the reactions and explain the principle involved in the assay of hydrogen peroxide.
b. What are radio-opaque contrast media? Give properties and uses of barium sulphate.
c. Define metabolic acidosis and metabolic alkalosis. Name the compounds used to treat them.
d. Write the role of Iodine in the body. Give storage condition and incompatibility of ferrous sulphate.
e. Mention different test for purity are performed on the substances. Explain any two test for purity.

Q 6. Solve any three:
a. Enlist the various counters used for measurement of radioactivity. Explain the construction and working of Geiger-Muller counter.
b. Discuss the principle and reactions involved in the limit test for arsenic IP.
c. Write two identification test for:
   i. Chloride ion   ii. Calcium ion
d. Classify the gastrointestinal agents with examples.
e. How physiological acid-base balance is maintained in the body? Explain respiratory mechanism.

Summer Examination 2012
D Pharm First Year
Pharmaceutical Chemistry I

Q 1. Answer any five:
a. Explain Arrhenius acid-base theory with examples. Discuss the limitations of Arrhenius acid-base theory.
b. Give synonyms for the following:
   i. Hydrochloric acid
   ii. Calcium hydroxide
   iii. Sodium hydroxide
   iv. Boric acid
c. Define buffers. Discuss the importance of buffers in pharmacy.
d. Give properties, uses, storage conditions and molecular formulas for dilute ammonia solution.
e. Define antioxidants and explain their mechanism of action.
f. Write molecular formula for the following:
   i. Sodium metabisulphite

ii. Phosphoric acid
   iii. Sodium thiosulphate
   iv. Potassium hydroxide
   g. Write uses, storage conditions and assay principle of ferrous sulphate.

Q 2. Answer any *three*:
   a. Classify the various gastrointestinal agents with examples.
   b. Discuss uses of the following:
      i. Milk of magnesia
      ii. Magnesium sulphate
      iii. Calcium carbonate
      iv. Sodium nitrite
   c. State the requirements for an ideal antacid. How is antacid property valuated?
   d. Define the term 'Achlorhydria'. Name the drug used for its treatment, mention its properties and molecular formula.
   e. What are anticaries agents? Discuss the role of fluoride as anticaries agent.

Q 3. Answer any *three*:
   a. Discuss the properties and uses of Dimethicone and Talc.
   b. Explain the mechanism of action of antimicrobial agents with examples.
   c. Give synonym, molecular formula, action and uses and storage conditions for chlorinated lime.
   d. Enlist various iodine preparations and explain the advantages of povidone-iodine solution.
   e. Discuss storage and labelling of the following:
      i. Nitrous oxide
      ii. Carbon dioxide

Q 4. Answer any *three*:
   a. Define astringents and discuss their uses.
   b. Define expectorants and emetics with examples. Discuss action and uses of ammonium chloride.
   c. Enlist various major extra- and intracellular electrolytes occurring in human body. Discuss the physiological role of potassium ions.
   d. Discuss the importance of ORS in physiological electrolyte imbalance.
   e. Write structural formula and uses of calcium gluconate. Why calcium gluconate is superior to calcium chloride?

Q 5. Answer any *three*:
a. How inadequate storage affect purity of pharmaceutical substance? Explain with two examples.
b. Explain principle involved in the limit test for iron IP.
c. Classify the antidotes with examples. Discuss cyanide poisoning along with its treatment.
d. Give two identification test for each:
   i. Chloride ion   ii. Calcium ion
e. Write therapeutic application of radio pharmaceuticals with examples.

Q 6. Answer any *three*:
a. Explain theory involved in the assay of sodium chloride with reactions.
b. Enlist various units used for measuring radioactivity. Write working of G.M. counter.
c. Discuss various methods for making permanent hard water soft.
d. Give synonyms for the following:
   i. Sodium potassium tartarate
   ii. Potassium aluminium sulphate
   iii. Calcium carbonate
   iv. Barium sulphate suspension.
e. Draw a well-labelled diagram of gutzeit apparatus.

Winter Examination 2012
D Pharm First Year
Pharmaceutical Chemistry I

Q 1. Answer any *five*:
a. Explain why glycerine is used in the assay of boric acid. Give reactions involved.
b. Discuss the various uses of radioisotopes in pharmacy.
c. Give uses and properties of ferrous sulphate and calcium carbonate.
d. Define buffers. Explain mechanism of action of buffers.
e. Explain Lowery-Bronsted theory with examples.
f. Name four official antioxidants.
g. Give synonyms and molecular formula for:
   i. Calcium hydroxide   ii. Hydrochloric acid.

Q 2. Answer any *three*:
a. Explain the physiological acid–base balance in the body.
b. Define and classify antidotes with examples.

c. Write properties and uses of:
   i. Talc
   ii. Kaolin
d. Explain with reactions principle involved in the assay of hydrogen peroxide solution.
e. Define the terms with examples:
   i. Lewis acid and Lewis base
   ii. Antiseptic and Disinfectant.

Q 3. Answer any *three*:
a. Explain the importance of "Combination antacid therapy".
b. Discuss the effect of impurities present in pharmaceuticals.
c. Discuss the biological effects of radiations on human body.
d. Name four official calcium compounds along with their molecular formula.
e. Mention uses of:
   i. Chlorinated lime
   ii. Selenium sulphide

Q 4. Answer any *three*:
a. Explain the principle along with reactions involved in iron limit test IP.
b. Define cathartics. Classify with examples.
c. Explain role of sodium ion as major extra-cellular electrolyte.
d. Define radio-opaque contrast media. Explain properties and uses of barium sulphate.
e. Discuss dehydration products of boric acid with reactions.

Q 5. Answer any *three*:
a. What are topical agents? Classify with examples.
b. Give storage and labelling for:
   i. Oxygen
   ii. Carbon dioxide
c. Give two identification tests for:
   i. Chloride
   ii. Calcium
d. Draw a well-labeled, neat diagram of Gutzeit apparatus.
e. Explain the importance of quality control in pharmacy.

Q 6. Answer any *three*:
a. Explain the role of fluoride ion in dental caries. Give properties and storage conditions for sodium fluoride and stannous fluoride.
b. Classify gastrointestinal agents with examples. Give uses of aluminum hydroxide gel and magnesium trisilicate.

148 Pharmaceutical Chemistry I

   c. Give synonyms for:
      i. Potassium aluminium sulphate.
      ii. Barium sulphate suspension
      iii. Potassium hydroxide
      iv. Antimony potassium tartarate
   d. Discuss the applications of astringents.
   e. Explain the principle involved in the limit test for lead IP along with the reactions.

Summer Examination 2013
D Pharm First Year
Pharmaceutical Chemistry I

Q 1. Attempt any *eight*:
   a. Explain acid-base as per Bronsted and Lowery theory.
   b. List some important antioxidants used in pharmaceutical formulations.
   c. Classify topical agents with examples.
   d. What are desensitizing agents?
   e. Give the different conditions under which oxygen is required to the body.
   f. What are respiratory stimulants?
   g. Give uses of ammonium chloride.
   h. Define and classify antidotes.
   i. Give formula for ORS.
   j. Enlist the official compounds of iron.
   k. Enlist various devices used in measurement of radiations.
   l. Define:
      i. Accuracy
      ii. Precision.

Q 2. Attempt any *four*:
   a. Give properties, storage and uses of Boric acid
   b. Give four ideal characteristics of an antacid. Describe importance of combination preparations of antacid.
   c. How will you treat cyanide poisoning using inorganic compounds?
   d. Enlist sodium chloride formulations used in electrolyte replacement therapy.
   e. Give formula, synonym, properties and uses of ferrous sulphate.
   f. Describe the limit test for iron.

Q 3. Attempt any *four*:
a. Define achlorhydria. Give properties, storage and uses of HCl.
b. State the properties and uses of:
   i. Calamine ii. Silicones.
c. What is the role of fluoride as anticaries agent?
d. What is metabolic acidosis and alkalosis?
e. Draw diagram of Gutzeit apparatus. Give the reactions involved in limit test of arsenic.
f. Give identification test for:
   i. Bicarbonates ii. Bromides.

Q 4. Attempt any *four*:
a. Give the mechanism by which antioxidants act and mention the properties of sulphur dioxide.
b. What are saline cathartics? Give properties and uses of magnesium sulphate.
c. Define antimicrobial agents. Explain mechanism by which they act.
d. Give the method of preparation, properties and uses of zinc chloride.
e. What is electrolyte combination therapy? Explain in detail.
f. Enlist official compounds of calcium. Give properties and uses of calcium gluconate.

Q 5. Attempt any *four*:
a. Define astringents. Give properties and uses of alum.
b. What is the role of oxygen in biological system?
c. Give synonym, formula, properties and uses of antimony potassium tartarate.
d. Draw a neat labelled diagram of Geiger-Muller counter. Give biological effects of radiation.
e. Give the principle, reactions and procedure involved in the limit test for sulphate.
f. Give identification tests for:
   i. Chloride ii. Calcium.

Q 6. Attempt any *four*:
a. Define buffer. Give mechanism of buffer action with suitable example.
b. Define protectives and adsorbents. Give synonym, properties and uses of bismuth subcarbonate.
c. Give different forms of sulphur. State properties and uses of selenium sulphide.
d. How the physiological acid–base balance of the body is maintained?

e. Give the labelling, storage and handling precautions in regard of radiopharmaceuticals. Explain properties and uses of Barium sulphate.
f. Write four important sources of impurities in pharmaceuticals with suitable examples.

Winter Examination 2013
D Pharm First Year
Pharmaceutical Chemistry I

Q 1. Solve any *five* of the following:
a. Define buffer solutions and list the important properties with examples.
b. Explain the principle behind limit test for sulphates with special reference to barium sulphate reagent as per I.P. 1985.
c. Define acid and base as per arrhenius concept and list the limitations.
d. Define antioxidants and give six important characteristics of an ideal antioxidant.
e. Give the molecular formula and uses of sodium nitrite and sodium thiosulphate.
f. Define and classify gastrointestinal agents with examples.
g. Define antacids and explain the rational behind the combination of antacid preparations with example.

Q 2. Solve any *three* of the following:
a. Describe the four mechanism of action of cathartics with examples.
b. Define and classify topical agents with examples.
c. What are antimicrobials and explain their three mechanism of action with examples.
d. Define astringent and explain their actions.
e. Give the synonyms for the following (any *four*):
   i. Chlorinated lime
   ii. Aqueous iodine
   iii. Borax
   iv. Magnesium sulphate
   v. Aluminium

Q 3. Solve any *three* of the following:
a. Give the molecular formula and uses of:
   i. Selenium sulphide
   ii. Zinc sulphate.

b. List the properties and uses for (any *two*)
   i. Hydrogen peroxide
   ii. Potassium permanganate
   iii. Titanium dioxide.
c. Describe the properties, uses, storage and incompatibilities of Iodine.
d. What are anticaries? Explain the role of fluorides in dental caries.
e. Name the methods for measurement of radioactivity and explain G.M. counter with sketch.

Q 4. Solve any *three* of the following:

a. Define desensitizing and polishing agent and examples of each with molecular formula.
b. Give storage conditions and uses for oxygen and nitrous oxide.
c. Define expectorants and respiratory stimulants. Explain properties and uses of potassium iodide.
d. What is milk alkali syndrome? List the important functions of calcium ion in the body.
e. Give the formula of ORS recommended by WHO and UNICEF and explain it with example.

Q 5. Solve any *three* of the following:

a. Define metabolic acidosis. Explain how acid–base balance of the body is maintained.
b. Define m Eq/l and calculate the number of mEq of sodium chloride in one liter of 0.85% W/V solution.
c. Explain hypo- and hyperkalemia and summarise the conditions.
d. Describe the role of iron or iodine in the body.
e. List the inherent drawbacks of iron compounds. Name the important iron compounds with special reference to doses which are required as per patient need.

Q 6. Solve any *three* of the following:

a. Define radiopharmaceuticals and contrast media. Give the applications of cobalt (^{60}Co) and sodium iodide (^{131}I).
b. Define and classify antidotes with examples.
c. Explain the principle involved in limit test for iron with reaction.
d. Draw a neat labelled diagram of "Gutzeit" apparatus as per I.P. and write the reactions involved in limit test for arsenic.
e. Give two identification test for (each):
   i. Chlorides
   ii. Barium.

Winter Examination 2014
D Pharm First Year
Pharmaceutical Chemistry I

Q 1. Answer any *five* of the following:
  a. Define and give examples of drug used as a:
     i. Achlorhydria   ii. Expectorants
     iii. Inhalants   iv. Desensitizing agents.
  b. Define antidotes. Classify antidotes with examples.
  c. Explain the mechanism of action of antimicrobial agents with example.
  d. Give molecular formula, action and uses and storage condition of sodium nitrite.
  e. State molecular formula for the followings:
     i. Stannous fluoride   ii. Silicone polymers
     iii. Magnesium sulphate iv. Alum.
  f. Explain principle involved in the limit test for iron with reactions.
  g. State two identification tests for:
     i. Chloride ions   ii. Sulphate ions.

Q 2. Attempt any *three*:
  a. Define buffers. Give types and mechanism of buffers with suitable examples.
  b. State the properties and uses of Talc and Kaolin.
  c. Define laxatives, classify them with examples.
  d. Define astringents and discuss their applications.
  e. Explain importance of ORS mixture; give details of three formulae of ORS.

Q 3. Attempt any *three*:
  a. Give synonyms of the followings (any *four*):
     i. Antimony potassium tartrate
     ii. Sublimed sulphur
     iii. Chlorinated lime
     iv. Barium sulphate
     v. Sodium hydroxide
     vi. Ferrous sulphate.
  b. Explain the various preparations of iodine.
  c. Define topical agent. Classify topical agents with examples.
  d. State the storage and uses for:
     i. Oxygen   ii. Carbon dioxide.
  e. Classify antacids with examples, give properties of ideal antacids.

Q 4. Attempt any *three*:
   a. Explain Arrhenius acid-base theory with examples, give limitation of Arrhenius theory.
   b. Explain biological effects of radiations.
   c. Draw well labeled diagram of the apparatus used in the limit test for arsenic.
   d. Mention different allotropic forms of sulphur give properties and uses of Selenium sulphide.
   e. Define anticaries and dentifrices. Explain role of fluoride as anticaries agent.

Q 5. Attempt any *three*:
   a. Name at least one inorganic compound for each class.
      i. Scabies   ii. Dental caries
      iii. Antioxidants   iv. Respiratory stimulants.
   b. Give applications of radioactive isotopes in pharmacy.
   c. State Bronsted and Lowry concept of acid and bases with examples, give uses of boric acid and calcium hydroxide.
   d. Classify the various gastrointestinal agents with examples.
   e. Describe the role of iodine in the body. Enlist the any two official compounds of calcium with molecular formula.

Q 6. Attempt any *three*:
   a. Explain the labeling, handling, storage, precautions of radioactive materials.
   b. Explain physiological acid–base balance in the body.
   c. Enlist various devices used for the measurement of radioactivity. Explain working with neat sketch diagram of Geiger-Muller counter.
   d. Define GIT protectives, with examples give properties and uses of any one of them.
   e. Define the terms:
      i. Contrast media   ii. Quality control
      iii. Accuracy and precision   iv. Radioactivity.

Summer Examination 2015
D Pharm First Year
Pharmaceutical Chemistry I

Q 1. Attempt any *eight* of the following:
   a. Define the term monograph. What are the content of monograph?
   b. Define acid and base as per Lewis concept.

c. Define the terms:
   i. Accuracy and precision
   ii. Antiseptic and disinfectant
d. Define Achlorhydria and give name of agent used in this condition along with its role.
e. State molecular formula and uses of:
   i. Chlorinated lime
   ii. Silver nitrate.
f. Describe the reaction of boric acid with glycerin.
g. Explain combination antacid preparations in short.
h. Define antacid. Write ideal properties of antacid.
i. State synonym of the following:
   i. Sodium hydroxide
   ii. Calcium hydroxide
j. Define radioactivity. Enlist units used for measuring radioactivity.
k. Write importance of quality control.
l. State molecular formula and uses of magnesium trisilicate.

Q 2. Attempt any *four* of the following:

a. Define antidote. Explain the role of antidote in cyanide poisoning.
b. Define topical agents. Classify topical agent with examples.
c. Write storage condition of:
   i. Oxygen
   ii. Hydrogen peroxide
d. Mention allotropic forms of sulphur and describe properties and uses of selenium sulphide.
e. Calculate the mEq of sodium chloride in one litre of 0.9% w/v solution.
f. Explain how physiological acid-base balance of body is maintained.

Q 3. Attempt any *four* of the following:

a. Draw a neat labelled diagram of Gutzeit test apparatus with all specification mention in LR 96.
b. Define expectorant and write properties and uses of ammonium chloride.
c. Write molecular formula and uses of: (any **two**)
   i. Talc
   ii. Hypophosphorus acid
   iii. Strontium chloride
d. Define inhalant. Write storage and uses of carbon dioxide.
e. Explain metabolic acidosis and alkalosis. Write the uses of potassium citrate.
f. Define protective. Write properties and uses of calamine.

Q 4. Attempt any *four* of the following:
a. Define laxative and classify with examples.
b. Write the principle and reaction involved in limit test for iron.
c. Name the compound used as:
   i. Scabicides
   ii. Antidandruff
   iii. Anticaries
d. Explain the construction and working of G.M. counter.
e. Describe the role of iron in human body and write their official preparations.
f. Enlist the various sources of impurities in pharmaceutical substances. Explain any two.

Q 5. Attempt any *four* of the following:
a. Define gastrointestinal agent. Classify gastrointestinal agent with examples.
b. Define astringent. Write the important uses of astringent.
c. Write the procedure of limit test for chloride as per I.P.
d. Define respiratory stimulant and write properties, uses of ammonium carbonate.
e. Why povidorie-iodine is preferred to over elemental iodine. Give its three properties and uses.
f. Write any one I.P. identification test for:
   i. Acetate
   ii. Bicarbonate
   iii. Chloride

Q 6. Attempt any *four* of the following:
a. Enlist official compound of calcium and write molecular formula, uses of calcium gluconate.
b. Define antioxidants. Classify antioxidants with suitable examples and write criteria for selection of inorganic antioxidants.
c. Define buffer and write role of buffer in pharmacy.
d. Define radioactivity. Write properties of alpha, beta and gamma radiation.
e. What is radio-opaque contrast media? Write properties and uses of barium sulphate.
f. Define replacement therapy. Give official preparation and uses of sodium chloride.

Winter Examination 2015
D Pharm First Year
Pharmaceutical Chemistry I

Q 1. Attempt any *five* of the following:
   a. Define respiratory stimulant. Write brief account on ammonium carbonate as a respiratory stimulant.
   b. What are anticaries agent? Give properties and uses of sodium fluoride.
   c. Give the identification tests with chemical reactions for the following ions/radicals: (any **two**)
      i. Acetates
      ii. Calcium
      iii. Bicarbonates
   d. Give the uses and storage and labelling of the following:
      i. Oxygen
      ii. Carbon dioxide
   e. Give the principle, reactions and procedure involved in limit test for chloride (I.P.).
   f. Describe properties, uses, synonym and formula of calcium gluconate.
   g. Describe the assay principle arid reactions of boric acid with glycerine.

Q 2. Attempt any *three* of the following:
   a. Draw a well-labelled diagram for Gutzeit test apparatus (I.P.) for arsenic impurity in pharmaceuticals.
   b. Give the deficiency, symptoms and properties of iodine.
   c. Give the synonym of:
      i. Precipitated sulphur
      ii. Stannous fluoride
      iii. Borax
      iv. Zinc sulphate.
   d. Write incompatibilities of the following:
      i. Iron salts
      ii. Calcium gluconate
   e. Give chemical formula, properties and uses for: (any **two**)
      i. Calcium carbonate
      ii. Sodium nitrite
      iii. Ferrous sulphate

Q 3. Attempt any *three* of the following:
a. Give the principle and reactions involved in limit test of iron (I.P.).
b. Define emetics. Give molecular formula, synonym, properties and uses of antimony potassium tartrate.
c. What is quality control? Stress out the importance of quality control in pharmaceutical industry.
d. What are antidotes? Classify antidotes with examples.
e. Give properties, uses, synonym and molecular formula of sodium hydroxide.

Q 4. Attempt any *three* of the following:
a. Enlist the various sources of impurities. Explain the source—"Raw materials" and "Storage condition".
b. Discuss the various uses of radioisotopes in pharmacy.
c. Give the molecular formula, method of preparation, properties and uses of ammonium chloride.
d. Define pharmacopoeia and monograph. What are the contents of monograph?
e. Define antioxidants and state properties, chemical formula and uses of sodium metabisulphite.

Q 5. Attempt any *three* of the following:
a. Explain the mechanism of action of antimicrobial agents.
b. Give the synonym, molecular formula, properties, preparation and uses of chlorinated lime.
c. How the acid-base balance of the body is maintained?
d. What are desensitizing agents? Give properties and uses of strontium chloride.
e. Enlist the various devices used in measurement of radioactivity. Draw a neat labelled diagram of "Geiger - Muller Counter".

Q 6. Attempt any *three* of the following:
a. Explain Arrhenius acid-base theory with examples.
b. What is ORS? Give the formula of ORS given by WHO and UNICEF.
c. Define "radio-opaque contract media", and give properties and uses of barium sulphate.
d. Give one medicinal use of: (i) Aluminium hydroxide gel, (ii) Magnesium sulphate (iii) Bismuth subcarbonate (iv) Selenium sulphide
e. Give the properties and uses of: (any **two**)
   i. Talc
   ii. Calamine
   iii. Potassium permanganate
   iv. Hydrogen peroxide

Summer Examination 2016
D Pharm First Year
Pharmaceutical Chemistry I

Q 1. Attempt any *eight* of the following:
  a. Define acid and base as per Lewis theory with examples.
  b. Discuss the uses of aluminium hydroxide gel and magnesium sulphate.
  c. Define the following terms:
   i. Achlorhydria
   ii. Gastrointestinal agents
  d. Give the synonym of:
   i. Sodium potassium tartrate
   ii. Zinc sulphate
  e. Write the properties and uses of silicone polymers.
  f. What are dentifrices? Write the storage condition of sodium fluoride.
  g. Give the incompatibilities of:
   i. Iodine
   ii. Silver nitrate
  h. Write the reaction involved in limit test of iron. What is the role of thioglycolic acid in iron limit test.
  i. Give the molecular formula of the following:
   i. Borax
   ii. Yellow mercuric oxide
  j. Name major intra and extracellular electrolytes.
  k. Define buffers. Enlist various buffers used in Pharmacy.
  l. Explain handling and storage of radioactive material.

Q 2. Attempt any *four* of the following:
  a. Give the properties and uses of calcium hydroxide.
  b. Define antioxidants. Write factors for the selection of suitable antioxidant.
  c. Write properties, uses and incompatibilities of sodium thiosulphate.
  d. Defme and classify antacids with suitable examples.
  e. Give the molecular formula of :
   i. Talc
   ii. Calamine
   iii. Chlorinated lime
  f. Discuss the term ORS with examples.

Q 3. Attempt any *four* of the following:
a. Write molecular formula, properties and uses of calcium carbonate.
b. State molecular formula, synonym and uses of sodium metabisulphite.
c. Define and classify topical agents with examples.
d. Name the inorganic pharmaceuticals used in the treatment of constipation. Write properties and uses of bismuth subcarbonate.
e. Befine the term anticaries agents and desensitising agents with example. What is dental fluorosis?
f. State molecular formula, properties and uses of calcium gluconate.

Q 4. Attempt any *four* of the following:
a. Mention molecular formula and uses of stannous fluoride and strontium chloride.
b. What are metabolic acidosis and metabolic alkalosis? Name two compounds used to treat metabolic acidosis.
c. Write the principle and procedure involved in the limit test for sulphate as per I.P. 1996.
d. Give the properties molecular formula and uses of ammonium chloride.
e. What are protectives and adsorbents. Give the classification and ideal properties of the same.
f. Discuss the properties and uses of potassium permanganate.

Q 5. Attempt any *four* of the following:
a. Discuss uses and storage condition of:
   i. Oxygen
   ii. Nitrous oxide
b. State the uses of :
   i. Sodium acetate
   ii. Potassium citrate
c. Give the molecular formula, uses and storage condition of ammonium carbonate.
d. Define mEq. Calculate the mEq of NaCl in one litre of 1.6% w/v of solution.
e. What are radiopharmaceuticals? Give the characteristics of alpha particles.
f. Name two official compounds of iron. Discuss the properties and uses of ferrous sulphate.

Q 6. Attempt any *four* of the following:
a. Define the term Curie and microCurie. Draw well-labelled diagram of G.M. counter.
b. Enlist different allotropic forms of sulfur. Explain properties and uses of precipitated sulfur.
c. Discuss the principle and reactions involved in the limit test for arsenic.
d. Give any two identification tests for the following: (any **two**)
   i. Carbonate
   ii. Acetate
   iii. Calcium
e. Define the following terms:
   i. Expectorant
   ii. Respiratory stimulants
   iii. Antidotes
   iv. Cathartics
f. Define the term impurity. Explain various sources of impurities present in pharamaceuticals.

Winter Examination 2016
D Pharm First Year
Pharmaceutical Chemistry I

Q 1. Attempt any *five* of the following:
a. Explain Bronsted Lowry theory of acids and bases with examples and give its advantages over Arrhenius theory.
b. What are topical antimicrobial agents? Classify them based on their mechanism of action.
c. Describe limit test for iron as per IP and give role of iron free citric acid and iron free ammonia in the test.
d. Define antioxidants. Enlist the criteria for selection of antioxidants.
e. Write chemical name and molecular formula for:
   i Epsom salt   iii. Rochelle salt
   ii Muriatic acid   iv. Precipitated chalk
f. Explain why antacids are given in combination.
g. Write uses of:
   i Selenium sulphide
   ii Boric acid
h. Define 'Astringents'. Discuss their uses.

Q 2. Attempt any *three* of the following:
a. Enlist the 'source of impurities in pharmaceuticals' and explain any two with examples.
b. Define 'hyperchlorhydria' and give its symptoms. Write the role of hydrochloric acid in stomach.
c. Give properties and uses of calamine and talc.
d. Define 'volume strength' and calculate volume strength of 27% w/v H_2O_2 solution.
e. What are ORS mixtures? Give composition of ORS mixtures recommended by WHO and UNICEF.

Q 3. Attempt any *three* of the following:
a. What is 'quality control'? Give its significance in pharmacy.
b. Write chemical properties and uses of potassium permaganate and hydrogen peroxide.
c. Give properties and uses of magnesium trisilicate and aluminium hydroxide.
d. What is 'slaked lime'? Give its properties uses and molecular formula.
e. Discuss mechanism of action of antoxidants. Give molecular formula of sodium thiosulphate and sodium nitrite.

Q 4. Attempt any *three* of the following:
a. Define the terms:
   i. Hyponatremia
   ii. Anticaries agents
   iii. Hyperkalemia
   iv. Desensitizers
b. Give uses, storage condition and labelling requirement of oxygen gas.
c. What is 'shadow meal'? Give its properties, uses and molecular formula.
d. Explain how dental caries are formed and give role of fluoride in prevention of dental caries.
e. Define antidotes and explain treatment of cyanide poisoning.

Q 5. Attempt any *three* of the following:
a. Write molecular formula and uses of ammonium chloride and sodium bicarbonate.
b. Give role of iron in body. Enlist four official iron compounds.
c. Define 'Respiratory stimulants'. Give chemical formula and properties of ammonium carbonate.
d. What are 'Expectorants'? Classify them. Give uses of potassium iodide.

e. Define 'metabolic acidosis' and 'metabolic' alkalosis. Give the name of compounds used for their treatment.

Q 6. Answer any *three* of the following:
a. Write two identification tests each for ammonium and carbonate ions with the reaction involved.
b. Enlist various applications of radiosotopes.
c. Classify gastrointestinal agents with examples.
d. Define 'half-life of radioisotopes explain the units 'curie' and 'Rad' used for measurement of radiation.
e. Write molecular formula of calcium gluconate. Write its uses and give reason why it is preferred over other calcium salts.

Summer Examination 2017
D Pharm First Year
Pharmaceutical Chemistry I

Q 1. Answer any *five* of the following:
a. Give synonyms and molecular formula for:
  i. Boric acid
  ii. Calcium hydroxide
b. Define and classify GI agents with example.
c. Explain Lewis acid-base theory with examples.
d. Define different terminologies as antimicrobial agents.
e. Discuss importance of radioisotopes in pharmacy.
f. Enlist four official antioxidants.
g. Define buffer. Explain importance of pharmaceutical buffer.
h. Why glycerin is used in assay of boric acid? Explain with reactions.

Q 2. Answer any *three* of the following:
a. Define and classify antidotes.
b. Give mechanism of action of antioxidants and mention the properties and uses of sodium thiosulphate.
c. Explain the reaction and principle behind limit test for chloride.
d. Discuss Arrhenius acid-base theory with example and list limitations for it.
e. Explain the role of sodium ions as major extracellular electrolyte.

Q 3. Answer any *three* of the following:
a. "Andtacids are preffered in combination therapy". Why?
b. Define achlorhydria. Explain acidifying agent with its formula and uses.

c. Enlist four official compounds of Iron.
d. Discuss any four different sources of impurities in pharmaceuticals.
e. Explain radio-opaque contrast media. Give properties and uses of barium sulphate.

Q 4. Answer any *three* of the following:
a. Name and draw well-labelled diagram of apparatus used in limit test for arsenic.
b. Define cathartics and mention different types of cathartics with examples.
c. Define topical agents. Discuss mechanism of action of topical antimicrobials.
d. Give properties and uses of:
   i. Sodium nitrite
   ii. Aluminium hydroxide gel
e. Give chemical formula for: (any **two**)
   i. Hypophosphorus acid
   ii. Calcium carbonate
   iii. Sodium hydroxide
   iv. Nitrous oxide

Q 5. Answer any *three* of the following:
a. What is oral rehydration salt (ORS)? Give details of formulations of it.
b. Give storage and labeling of:
   i. Oxygen
   ii. Carbon dioxide
c. Explain the following term with examples:
   i. Anticaries agents
   ii. Desensitising agents
d. Discuss the applications of astringents. Give properties of alum.
e. Explain the reaction and principle involved in the assay of hydrogen peroxide.

Q 6. Answer any *three* of the following:
a. Explain physiological acid-base balance.
b. Define expectorant. Give properties and uses of ammonium chloride.
c. Give properties and uses of calcium hydroxide and ferrous sulphate.
d. Explain the principle and reaction involved in iron limit test I.P.
e. Give two identification tests for: (any **two**)
   i. Chloride ion
   ii. Calcium ion
   iii. Sodium ion
   iv. Acetate ion